THE COMPLETE PSORIASIS DIET FOR BEGINNERS

2024 EDITION

Nourishing Recipes to Soothe Your Skin and Boost Your Well-Being

VAKARE RIMKUTE

This Cookbook Belong to:

Name: _____

Copyright © 2024 by Vakare Rimkute

All rights reserved. No part of this publication may be reproduced, distributed, or transmitted in any form or by any means, including photocopying, recording, or other electronic or mechanical methods, without the prior written permission of the publisher, except in the case of brief quotations embodied in critical reviews and certain other noncommercial uses permitted by copyright law.

⚠ Disclaimer

The recipes and information presented in this cookbook are intended for general informational purposes only. While Vakare Rimkute has made every effort to ensure the accuracy and completeness of the content, they make no representations or warranties of any kind, express or implied, about the suitability or applicability of the recipes for any purpose .

Introduction to Psoriasis

Psoriasis is more than just a skin condition; it's a daily battle that affects both the body and the spirit. For those diagnosed with psoriasis, the journey is often fraught with challenges, from the physical discomfort of flare-ups to the emotional toll of navigating social situations. But amidst the struggle, there is hope, resilience, and a path to wellness that begins with understanding and nurturing your body from within.

This cookbook, "**Psoriasis Diet for Beginners,**" is born out of compassion and a deep desire to empower you on your journey to better health. It is a collection of recipes thoughtfully crafted to nourish your body and soothe your skin. Each dish is designed with ingredients known to combat inflammation and promote skin health, helping you take control of your condition one meal at a time.

Living with psoriasis can sometimes feel isolating, but remember, you are not alone. Countless others understand your journey, and have walked the same path and found solace in the power of nutrition. This book is not just about food; it's about building a community of support and encouragement, a testament to the strength and resilience that lies within each of us.

As you turn the pages of this cookbook, you'll find more than just recipes. You'll discover tips for managing your condition, advice for creating a psoriasis-friendly pantry, and stories from others who have found relief and joy in eating well. These pages are filled with hope, practical wisdom, and the promise of a healthier, happier you.

Embrace this journey with an open heart and a courageous spirit. The road to wellness is a marathon, not a sprint, but every step you take is a victory.

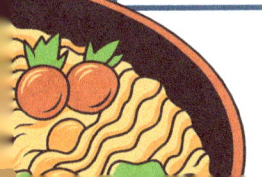
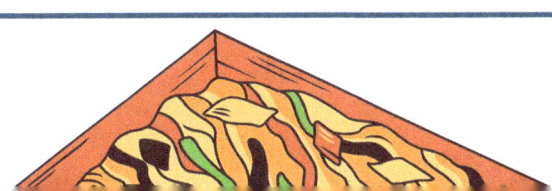

Celebrate your progress, no matter how small, and trust that with each nutritious meal, you give your body the tools it needs to heal and thrive.

Here's to new beginnings, to vibrant health, and to the strength that comes from within. May this cookbook be your companion, your guide, and your source of encouragement as you embark on this transformative journey. Remember, the power to change your health is in your hands, and with every mindful bite, you are taking a bold step towards a brighter, healthier future.

You are stronger than you know, and this is just the beginning. Let's take this journey together, one delicious recipe at a time.

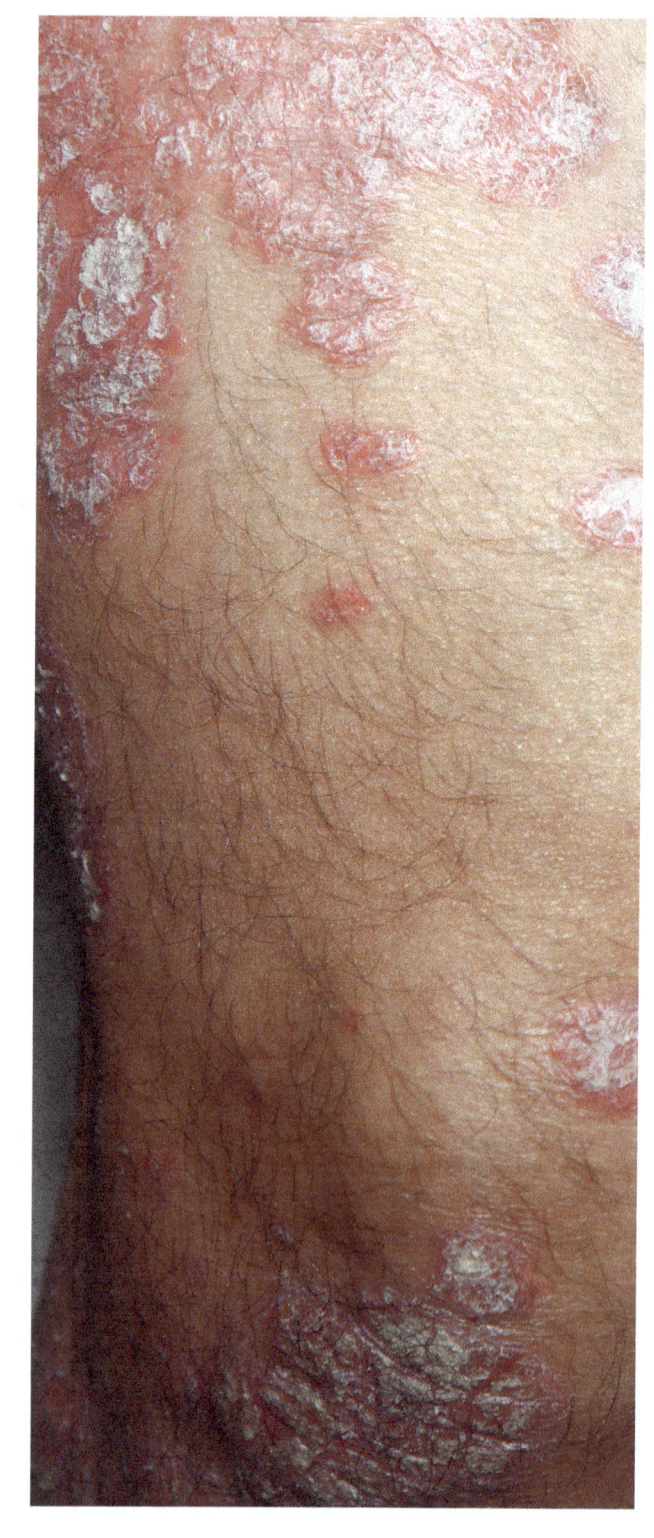

TABLE OF Content

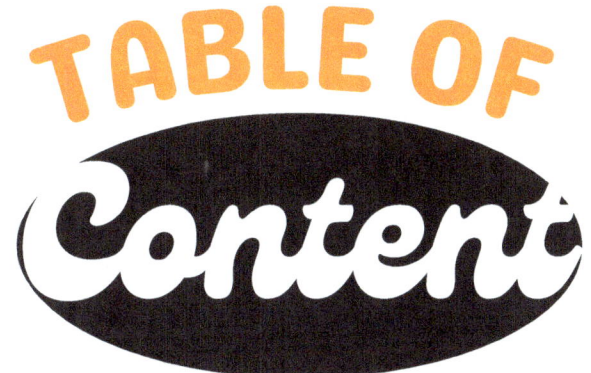

i. **Introduction to Psoriasis**

1. **Understanding Psoriasis**
2. **Breakfasts**
3. **Lunches**
4. **Dinners**
5. **Snacks and Sides**
6. **Digestive Health and Gut Support**
7. **Delicious Desserts**
8. **Beverages for Wellness**
9. **Shopping List**
10. **Natural Remedies and Supplements**
11. **Sleep Hygiene and Skin Health**

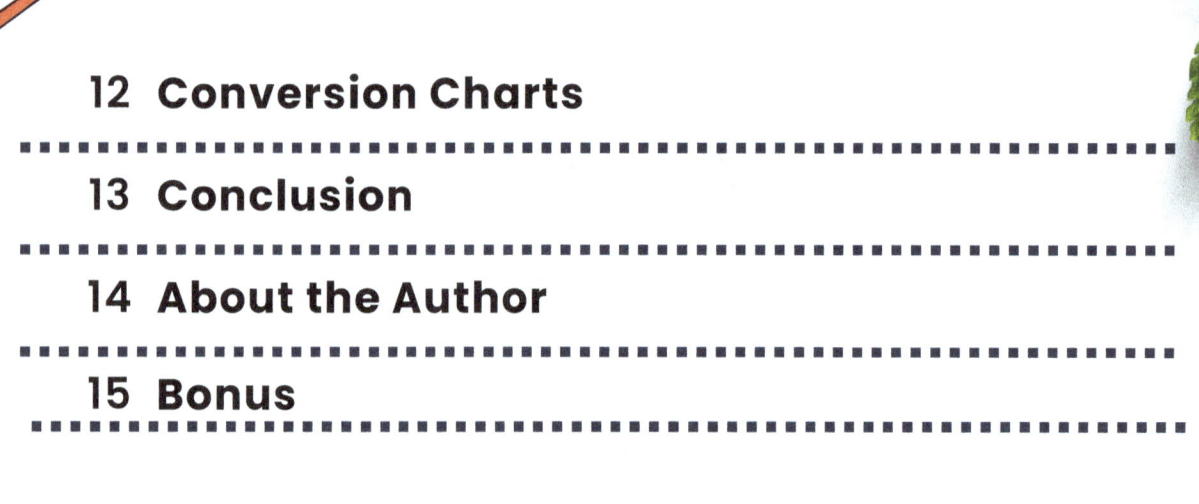

12	Conversion Charts
13	Conclusion
14	About the Author
15	Bonus

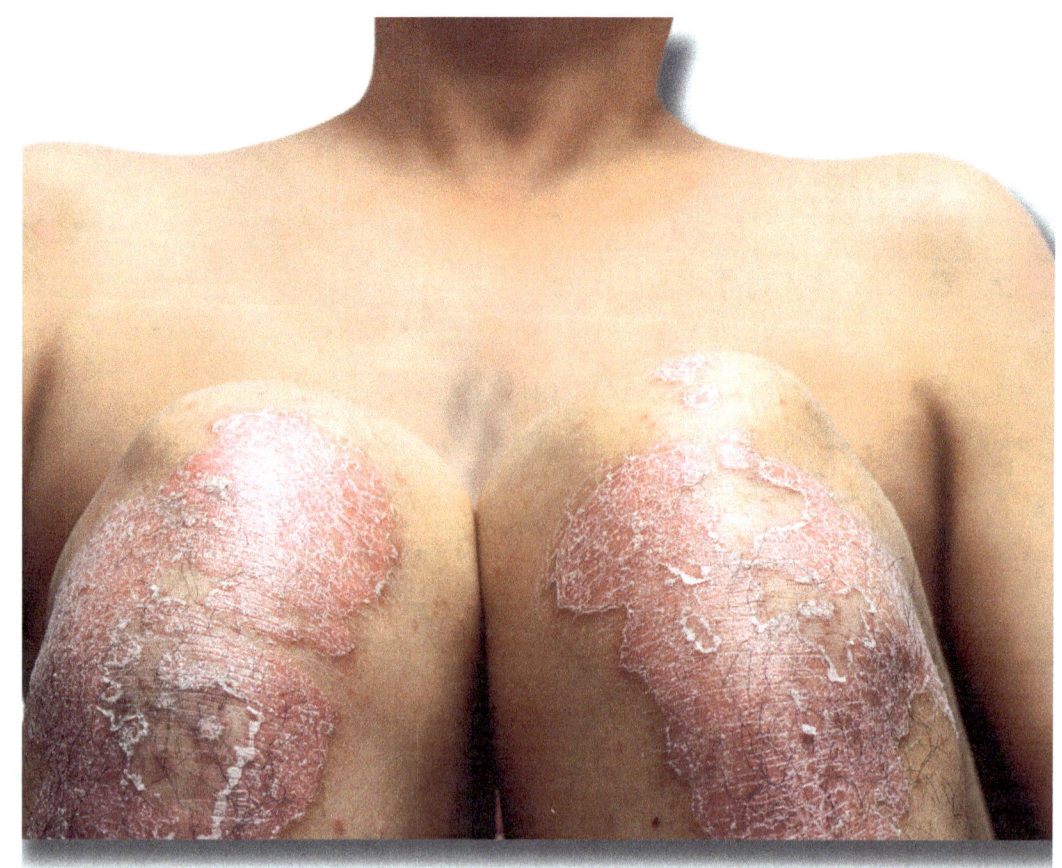

CHAPTER 1

Understanding Psoriasis

What is Psoriasis?

Psoriasis is a chronic autoimmune condition that causes the rapid buildup of skin cells, leading to scaling on the skin's surface. This buildup of cells causes scaling and red patches that can be itchy and sometimes painful. Psoriasis is a long-lasting disease that typically goes through cycles, flaring for a few weeks or months, then subsiding for a while or going into remission.

Types of Psoriasis

1. Plaque Psoriasis (Psoriasis Vulgaris)
- **Description**: The most common form, affects about 80-90% of people with psoriasis.
- **Symptoms**: Raised, inflamed, red lesions covered with silvery white scales. These plaques can be itchy and painful and may crack and bleed.
- **Common Areas**: Elbows, knees, scalp, and lower back.

2. Guttate Psoriasis
- **Description**: Often starts in childhood or young adulthood.
- **Symptoms**: Small, dot-like lesions that can appear suddenly. These lesions are usually not as thick as plaque psoriasis.
- **Common Triggers:** Often triggered by a bacterial infection such as strep throat.

3. Inverse Psoriasis
- **Description**: Affects skin folds and areas where skin rubs against skin.
- **Symptoms**: Bright red, shiny lesions that appear smooth and are not scaly. The affected areas can be very irritated and painful.
- **Common Areas**: Under the breasts, in the groin, around the buttocks, and under the arms.

4. Pustular Psoriasis
- **Description**: Characterized by white pustules (blisters of noninfectious pus) surrounded by red skin.
- **Symptoms**: The pustules can form in large areas or be localized to specific areas such as the hands and feet (palmoplantar pustulosis).
- **Forms**: It can be generalized, covering large areas of the body, or localized.

5. Erythrodermic Psoriasis
- **Description**: The least common but most severe form of psoriasis.
- **Symptoms**: Widespread, fiery redness over most of the body. It can cause severe itching, pain, and peeling of the skin in large sheets.
- **Triggers**: Often triggered by severe sunburn, infection, certain medications, or abrupt withdrawal from systemic psoriasis treatment.

6. Nail Psoriasis
- **Description**: Affects the nails of fingers and toes.
- **Symptoms**: Pitting, discolouration, thickening of the nails, and separation of the nail from the nail bed (onycholysis). Nails may also crumble.

7. Scalp Psoriasis
- **Description**: Specifically affects the scalp.
- **Symptoms**: Red patches covered with silvery scales, dandruff-like flaking, and possible hair loss. It can extend beyond the hairline onto the forehead, the back of the neck, and around the ears.

8. Psoriatic Arthritis
- **Description**: A type of arthritis that affects some people with psoriasis.
- **Symptoms**: Joint pain, stiffness, and swelling, which can affect any joint. It can also cause swelling of the fingers and toes (dactylitis) and back pain (spondylitis).

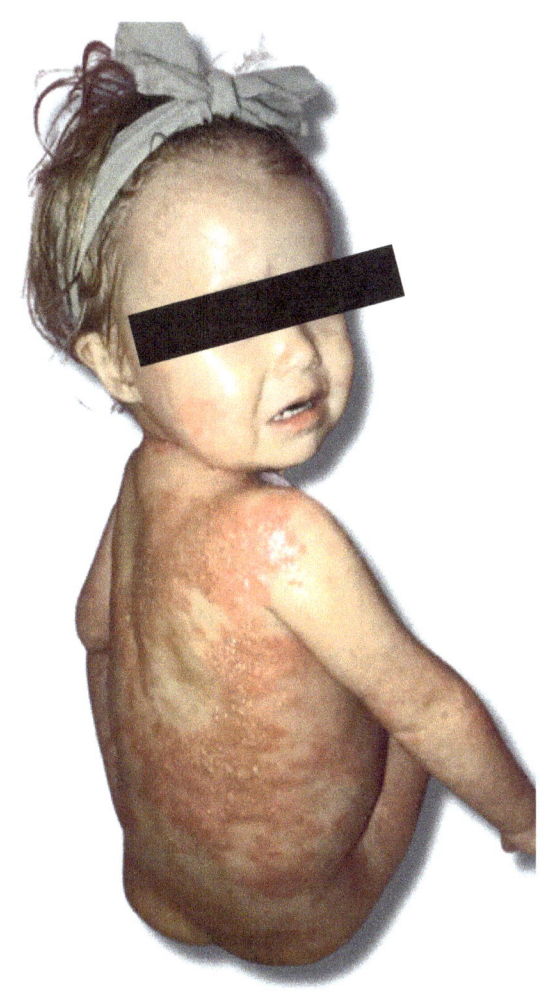

Causes of Psoriasis

1. **Genetic Factors**
   - **Family History**: Psoriasis tends to run in families. If one or both parents have psoriasis, there is a higher chance that their children may develop the condition.
   - **Genetic Mutations**: Certain genetic mutations are associated with psoriasis. These mutations can affect the immune system and skin cell production.

2. **Immune System**
   - **Autoimmune Response:** Psoriasis is an autoimmune disorder where the immune system mistakenly attacks healthy skin cells. This leads to an overproduction of skin cells, resulting in the characteristic scales and plaques.
   - **Inflammation:** Immune system activity triggers inflammation, which contributes to the redness and swelling seen in psoriasis lesions.

3. **Environmental Triggers**
   - **Infections**: Certain infections, such as strep throat, can trigger or exacerbate psoriasis, particularly guttate psoriasis.
   - **Skin Injuries:** Cuts, scrapes, bug bites, or severe sunburns can trigger a psoriasis outbreak at the site of the injury, known as the Koebner phenomenon.

4. **Lifestyle Factors**
   - **Stress**: High-stress levels can trigger or worsen psoriasis flare-ups. Stress management techniques can help reduce the frequency and severity of outbreaks.
   - **Diet**: While diet alone does not cause psoriasis, certain foods can trigger or exacerbate symptoms in some people. A diet high in anti-inflammatory foods may help manage symptoms.

5. **Medications**
   - **Certain Drugs:** Some medications can trigger or worsen psoriasis. These include lithium (used to treat bipolar disorder), antimalarial drugs, some blood pressure medications (beta-blockers), and corticosteroids (especially when they are abruptly discontinued).

6. **Lifestyle Factors**
   - **Smoking**: Smoking is a known risk factor for developing psoriasis and can worsen the severity of the condition.
   - **Alcohol**: Heavy alcohol consumption can trigger psoriasis flare-ups and interfere with treatment effectiveness.

Importance of Diet in Managing Psoriasis

1. Reducing Inflammation

Psoriasis is an inflammatory condition, and diet can either exacerbate or mitigate inflammation.

- **Anti-Inflammatory Foods:** Incorporate foods rich in antioxidants and omega-3 fatty acids, which help reduce inflammation. These include:
    - **Fruits and Vegetables:** Leafy greens, berries, citrus fruits, and colourful vegetables.
    - **Fatty Fish:** Salmon, mackerel, and sardines.
    - **Nuts and Seeds**: Almonds, walnuts, flaxseeds, and chia seeds.
    - **Healthy Fats:** Olive oil and avocados.
- **Avoiding Pro-Inflammatory Foods**: Reduce intake of foods that can increase inflammation, such as:
    - **Processed Foods:** High in trans fats and refined sugars.
    - **Red and Processed Meats:** These can contribute to inflammation.
    - **Sugary Snacks and Beverages**: High sugar content can trigger inflammatory responses.

2. Supporting the Immune System

Psoriasis is an autoimmune disorder, so maintaining a healthy immune system is crucial.

- **Nutrient-rich foods:** Vitamins and minerals are essential for immune function and skin health. Focus on:
    - **Vitamin D**: Found in fatty fish, and fortified foods, and produced by the body when exposed to sunlight.
    - **Vitamin A**: Found in leafy greens, carrots, and sweet potatoes.
    - **Vitamin E:** Found in nuts, seeds, and green leafy vegetables.
    - Zinc and Selenium: Found in nuts, seeds, and whole grains.
- **Identifying and Avoiding Triggers:** Some people with psoriasis may have specific food sensitivities. Common triggers include:
    - **Gluten:** For those with gluten sensitivity.
    - **Dairy Products:** Can be inflammatory for some individuals.
    - **Nightshade Vegetables:** Such as tomatoes, potatoes, and eggplants, which may trigger symptoms in some people.

3. Weight Management

Maintaining a healthy weight can reduce the severity of psoriasis symptoms and the risk of associated conditions such as psoriatic arthritis.

- **Balanced Diet:** Emphasize whole foods, lean proteins, and healthy fats.
- **Portion Control:** Avoid overeating and focus on balanced meals to prevent weight gain.
- **Regular Physical Activity:** Combine a healthy diet with regular exercise for optimal weight management.

4. Promoting Gut Health

A healthy gut microbiome can influence immune system function and inflammation.

- **Probiotics:** Include fermented foods like yoghurt, kefir, sauerkraut, and kimchi to support gut health.
- **Fiber-Rich Foods:** Whole grains, fruits, vegetables, and legumes promote a healthy gut microbiome.

5. Hydration

Proper hydration is essential for overall health and skin hydration.

- **Water Intake:** Aim to drink plenty of water throughout the day to keep the skin hydrated and reduce dryness.
- **Limiting Alcohol:** Alcohol can dehydrate the body and trigger psoriasis flare-ups in some individuals.

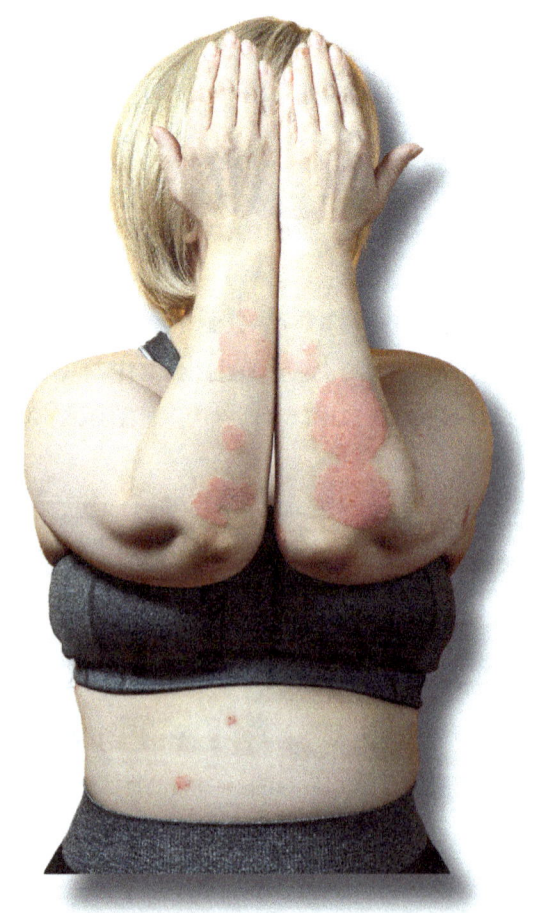

Foods to Avoid

Processed Foods

- **Examples**: Packaged snacks, fast food, sugary cereals, and ready-to-eat meals.
- **Impact**: Processed foods are often high in trans fats, refined sugars, and artificial additives, which can increase inflammation and worsen psoriasis symptoms.

Red and Processed Meats

- **Examples**: Beef, pork, bacon, sausages, and deli meats.
- **Impact**: These meats contain saturated fats and can produce inflammatory chemicals (arachidonic acid) that may trigger or aggravate psoriasis.

Dairy Products

- **Examples**: Milk, cheese, butter, and yoghurt.
- **Impact**: Dairy can be inflammatory for some individuals. The proteins in dairy products (casein and whey) may trigger immune responses that worsen psoriasis symptoms.

Gluten

- **Examples**: Wheat, barley, rye, and foods made from these grains like bread, pasta, and pastries.
- **Impact**: Gluten sensitivity or celiac disease can exacerbate psoriasis symptoms in some individuals. Gluten can cause inflammation and trigger immune responses.

Nightshade Vegetables

- **Examples**: Tomatoes, potatoes, eggplants, and bell peppers.
- **Impact**: These vegetables contain solanine, which can trigger inflammation and worsen psoriasis symptoms in some people. Sensitivity to nightshades varies among individuals.

Sugary Foods and Beverages

- **Examples**: Sodas, candy, desserts, and sweetened beverages.
- **Impact**: High sugar intake can lead to increased inflammation and weight gain, both of which can aggravate psoriasis symptoms. Sugary foods can also cause spikes in blood sugar levels, potentially impacting immune function.

Alcohol

- **Examples**: Beer, wine, spirits, and cocktails.
- **Impact**: Alcohol can dehydrate the body and skin, trigger immune responses, and increase inflammation. It can also interfere with psoriasis medications and treatments.

Fried and Fatty Foods

- **Examples**: Fried chicken, french fries, doughnuts, and other deep-fried items.
- **Impact**: These foods are typically high in trans fats and unhealthy oils, which can promote inflammation and negatively impact psoriasis.

Refined Carbohydrates

- **Examples**: White bread, white rice, pastries, and other refined grain products.
- **Impact**: Refined carbohydrates can cause spikes in blood sugar levels, leading to increased inflammation and potentially worsening psoriasis symptoms.

Mint and Mint-Flavored Products

- **Impact**: Mint can relax the LES, increasing the risk of acid reflux.
- **Examples**: Peppermint, spearmint, mint tea, and mint-flavored candies.

Tips for Avoiding Trigger Foods

- **Read Labels**: Check ingredient lists for hidden sources of gluten, dairy, and added sugars.
- **Cook at Home**: Preparing meals at home allows you to control ingredients and avoid harmful additives.
- **Choose Whole Foods**: Opt for whole grains, fresh fruits and vegetables, lean proteins, and healthy fats.
- **Experiment with Alternatives:** Find substitutes for common trigger foods, such as almond milk for dairy, or gluten-free grains like quinoa and brown rice.
- **Monitor Reactions:** Keep a food diary to track what you eat and how your psoriasis responds. This can help identify specific triggers.

Foods to Include

Fruits and Vegetables

- **Examples**: Berries, oranges, apples, carrots, spinach, kale, broccoli, and bell peppers.
- **Impact**: Rich in antioxidants, vitamins, and fibre, fruits and vegetables help reduce inflammation, support the immune system, and improve skin health.

Fatty Fish

- **Examples**: Salmon, mackerel, sardines, and anchovies.
- **Impact**: High in omega-3 fatty acids, which have anti-inflammatory properties that can help reduce psoriasis symptoms.

Nuts and Seeds

- **Examples**: Walnuts, flaxseeds, chia seeds, and almonds.
- **Impact**: Provide healthy fats, antioxidants, and omega-3 fatty acids that help reduce inflammation and support skin health.

Whole Grains

- **Examples**: Brown rice, quinoa, oatmeal, and whole wheat.
- **Impact**: Rich in fiber and nutrients, whole grains help regulate blood sugar levels and may reduce inflammation.

Lean Proteins

- **Examples**: Chicken, turkey, tofu, and legumes.
- **Impact**: Provide essential amino acids for overall health and help maintain muscle mass without contributing to inflammation.

Healthy Fats

- **Examples:** Olive oil, avocado, and coconut oil.
- **Impact**: Contains monounsaturated and polyunsaturated fats that can help reduce inflammation and support skin hydration.

Herbs and Spices

- **Examples**: Turmeric, ginger, garlic, and cinnamon.
- **Impact**: Have anti-inflammatory and antioxidant properties that can help manage psoriasis symptoms. Turmeric and ginger, in particular, contain compounds that may reduce inflammation.

Fermented Foods

- **Examples**: Yogurt (with live cultures), kefir, sauerkraut, and kimchi.
- **Impact**: Contains probiotics that support gut health and can influence immune function and inflammation positively.

Legumes

- **Examples**: Lentils, chickpeas, and black beans.
- **Impact**: High in fibre and protein, legumes help stabilize blood sugar levels and provide essential nutrients.

Green Tea

- **Examples**: Regular green tea or matcha.
- **Impact**: Contains antioxidants and polyphenols that have anti-inflammatory effects and may help reduce psoriasis symptoms.

Tips for Incorporating These Foods

- **Balanced Meals:** Aim to include a variety of these foods in each meal to ensure a balance of nutrients.
- **Colourful Plates:** Fill your plate with a rainbow of fruits and vegetables to maximize your intake of antioxidants and vitamins.
- **Healthy Cooking Methods**: Use methods like grilling, baking, steaming, or sautéing with healthy oils to prepare meals.
- **Experiment with Recipes:** Try new recipes that incorporate these beneficial foods to keep your diet varied and interesting.

BASIC INGREDIENT

Spinach	Olive oil	Barley
Kale	Avocado	Oats
Blueberries	Turmeric	Whole Wheat
Strawberries	Ginger	Turkey
Salmon	Greek yogurt	Lentils
Mackerel	Kefir	Coconut Oil
Almonds	Swiss Chard	Garlic
Walnuts	Arugula	Cinnamon
Flaxseeds	Raspberries	Sauerkraut
Chia seeds	Blackberries	Kimchi
Brown rice	Sardines	Sweet Potatoes
Quinoa	Trout	Carrots
Chicken breast	Sunflower Seeds	Broccoli
Tofu		

When to see a Doctor

Seeing a doctor for psoriasis is important if you notice new or <ins>worsening symptoms,</ins> such as expanding patches or increased severity. Severe flare-ups that cause significant discomfort or interfere with daily life also warrant a visit to ensure effective management. If your psoriasis affects large areas or sensitive regions like the <ins>face or genitals</ins>, specialized treatment may be needed.

You should also consult a doctor if your current treatment isn't providing relief or if you experience side effects. Signs of infection in psoriasis lesions, such as r<ins>edness, swelling, or pus,</ins> should be addressed to prevent complications. <ins>Joint pain, stiffness, or swelling could indicate psoriatic arthritis,</ins> which requires timely treatment to avoid joint damage.

If psoriasis is impacting your mental health, causing stress or depression, it's important to seek help. <ins>Pregnant or breastfeeding</ins> individuals should consult a healthcare provider to adjust treatments safely. Regular check-ups are crucial for monitoring your condition and adjusting your treatment plan as needed to ensure optimal care and management.

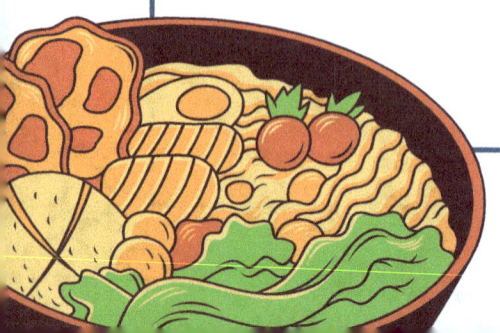
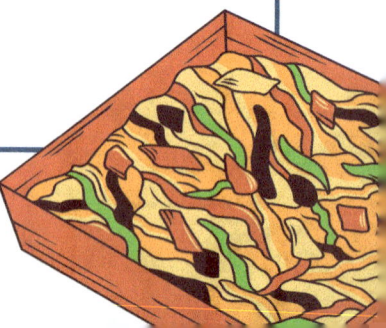

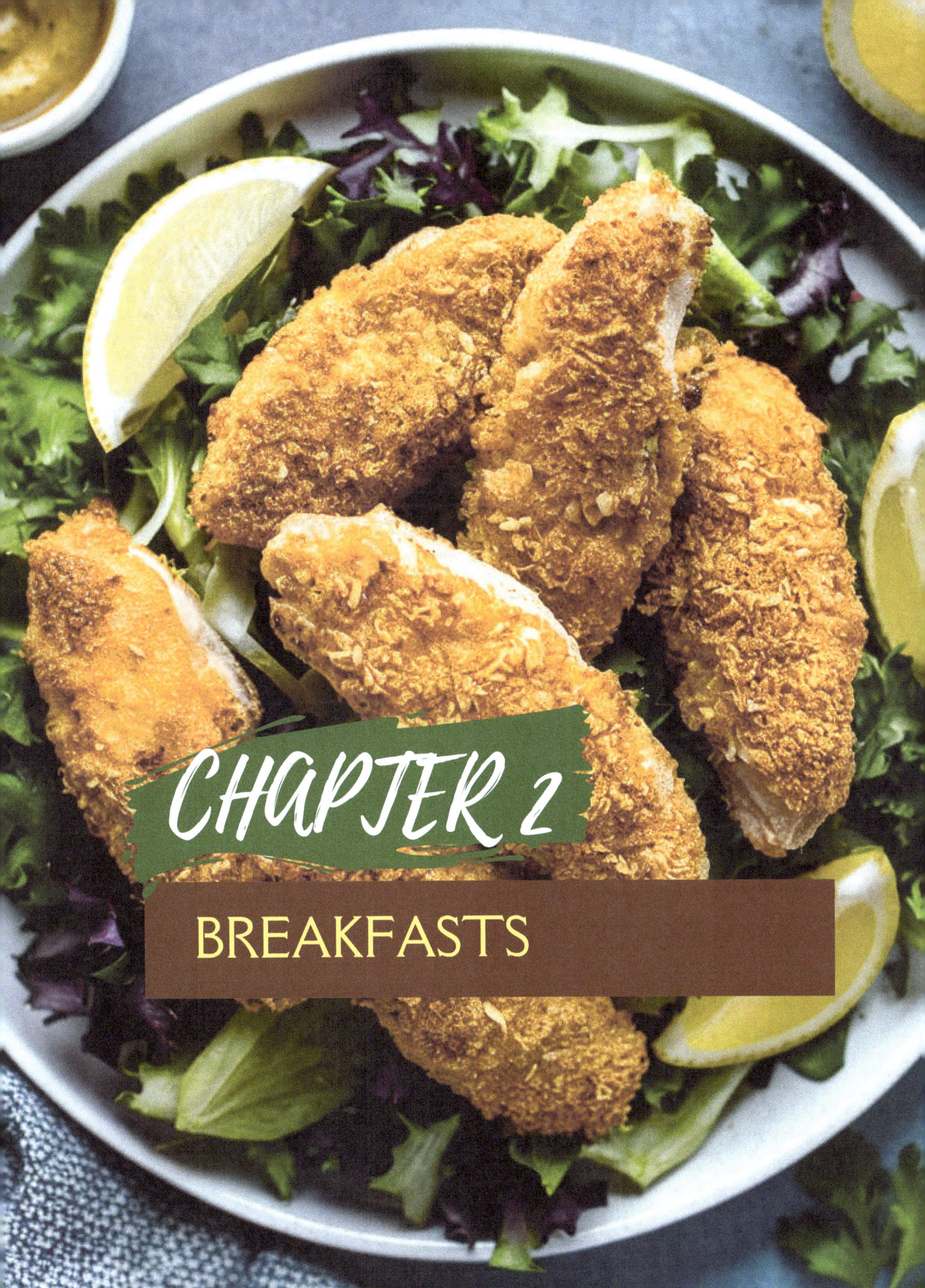

CHAPTER 2

BREAKFASTS

SPINACH AND MUSHROOM FRITTATA

Ingredients

- 1 cup fresh spinach, chopped
- 1 cup mushrooms, sliced
- 6 large eggs
- 1/4 cup milk (dairy or non-dairy)
- 1/2 cup shredded cheese (optional, can use dairy-free cheese)
- 1 small onion, finely chopped
- 1 clove garlic, minced
- Salt and pepper to taste
- 1 tablespoon olive oil

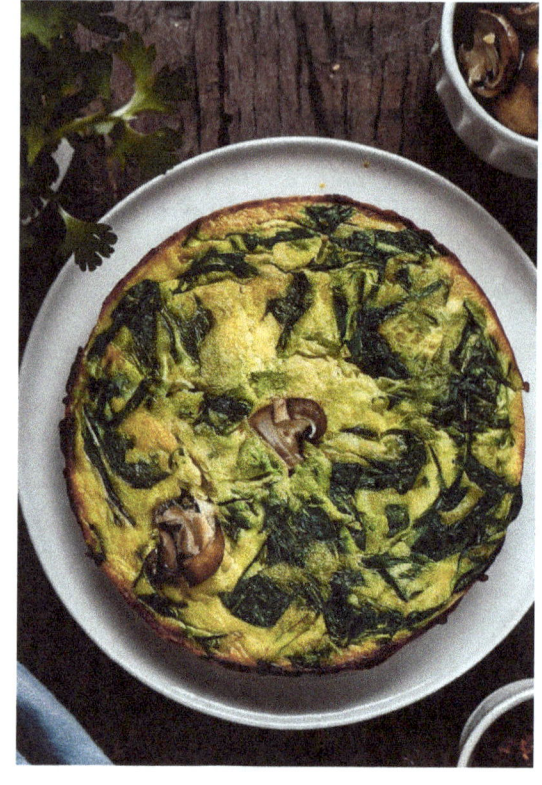

Instructions

- Preheat your oven to 375°F (190°C).
- In a large oven-safe skillet, heat the olive oil over medium heat.
- Add the chopped onion and garlic, sauté until fragrant and the onion is translucent, about 2-3 minutes.
- Add the sliced mushrooms to the skillet, cook until they release their moisture and start to brown, about 5 minutes.
- Add the chopped spinach to the skillet and cook until wilted, about 1-2 minutes.
- In a mixing bowl, whisk together the eggs, milk, salt, and pepper.
- Pour the egg mixture over the vegetables in the skillet. If using, sprinkle the shredded cheese evenly over the top.
- Cook on the stove for about 2-3 minutes until the edges start to set.
- Transfer the skillet to the preheated oven and bake for 10-12 minutes, or until the frittata is fully set and lightly golden on top.
- Remove from the oven, let it cool slightly, then slice into wedges and serve.

 Preparation Time : 10 min

 Total Time : 25 min

 Servings : 4

Nutritional Info

- Calories: 180
- Protein: 12g
- Fat: 12g
- Carbohydrates: 5g
- Fiber: 1g

SWEET POTATO AND KALE HASH

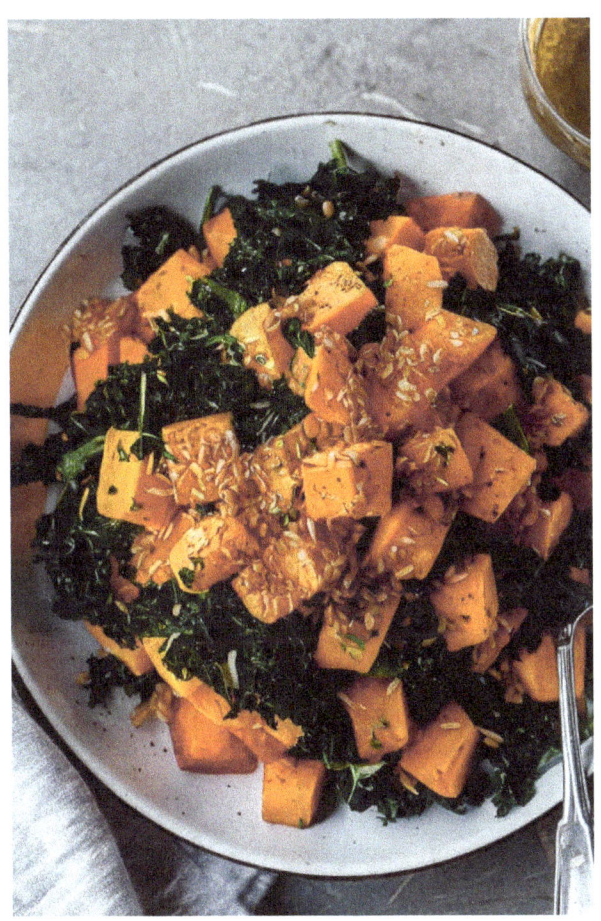

Ingredients

- 2 medium sweet potatoes, peeled and diced
- 1 bunch kale, stems removed and leaves chopped
- 1 onion, diced
- 2 garlic cloves, minced
- 1 tablespoon olive oil
- Salt and pepper, to taste

Instructions

- Heat olive oil in a large skillet over medium heat.
- Add onion and garlic, and sauté until onion is translucent.
- Add sweet potatoes and cook, stirring occasionally, until they start to soften, about 10 minutes.
- Stir in kale and cook until wilted.
- Season with salt and pepper.
- Serve hot.

 Preparation Time : 10 min

 Total Time : 30 min

 Servings : 4

Nutritional Info

- Calories: 180
- Fat: 4g
- Carbohydrates: 35g
- Fiber: 5g
- Protein: 3g

AVOCADO TOAST WITH POACHED EGG

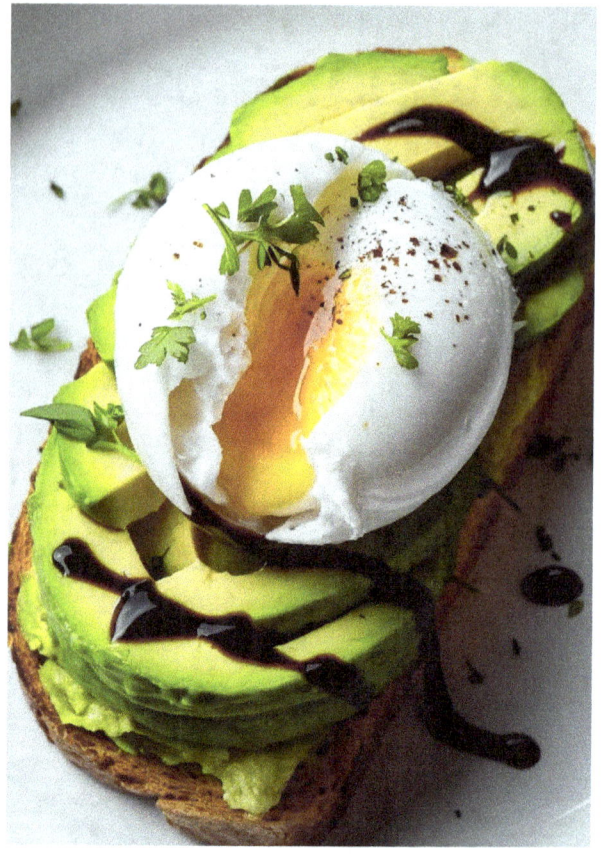

Ingredients

- 1 slice of whole grain bread
- 1/2 ripe avocado
- 1 egg
- Salt and pepper to taste
- Optional toppings: red pepper flakes, chopped chives.

Instructions

- Fill a small saucepan with water and bring it to a simmer.
- Crack the egg into a small bowl or cup.
- Create a gentle whirlpool in the water and carefully slide the egg into the center.
- Cook for about 3-4 minutes for a soft yolk, or longer for a firmer yolk.
- Remove the egg with a slotted spoon and place it on a paper towel to drain.
- While the egg is poaching, cut the avocado in half and remove the pit.
- Scoop out the flesh into a bowl and mash it with a fork.
- Toast the bread until golden brown and crispy.
- Spread the mashed avocado evenly onto the toasted bread.
- Place the poached egg on top.
- Season with additional salt and pepper if desired.
- Add any optional toppings like red pepper flakes, chopped chives, or a squeeze of lemon juice.
- Serve the avocado toast immediately and enjoy!

 Preparation Time : 5 min

 Total Time : 10 min

 Servings : 1

Nutritional Info

- Calories: 300 kcal
- Protein: 10g
- Fat: 20g
- Carbohydrates: 25g
- Fiber: 10g

TURMERIC AND GINGER SMOOTHIE

Ingredients

- 1 ripe banana
- 1 cup coconut milk (or any milk of your choice)
- 1/2 teaspoon ground turmeric
- 1/2 teaspoon grated ginger
- 1 tablespoon honey (optional, adjust to taste)
- Handful of ice cubes

Instructions

- Peel and chop the banana.
- Add all ingredients to a blender.
- Blend until smooth and creamy.
- Taste and adjust sweetness if necessary by adding more honey.
- Serve immediately in glasses.

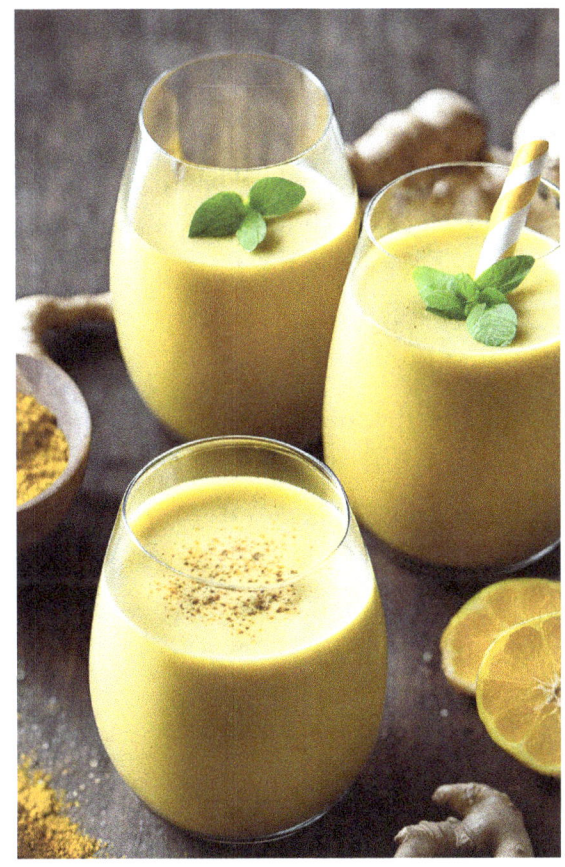

Preparation Time : 5 min

Total Time : 5 min

Servings : 2

Nutritional Info

- Calories: 120 kcal
- Fat: 6g
- Carbohydrates: 20g
- Protein: 1g
- Fiber: 3g

CHIA SEED BREAKFAST PUDDING

Ingredients

- 2 tablespoons chia seeds
- 1/2 cup almond milk (or any milk of your choice)
- 1/2 teaspoon vanilla extract
- 1 tablespoon honey or maple syrup (optional)
- Fresh fruits (such as berries, sliced banana, or mango) for topping
- Nuts or seeds for topping (such as sliced almonds, chopped walnuts, or pumpkin seeds)

Instructions

- In a bowl or jar, combine chia seeds, almond milk, vanilla extract, and honey or maple syrup (if using). Stir well to combine.
- Cover the bowl or jar and refrigerate overnight, or for at least 4 hours, to allow the chia seeds to absorb the liquid and thicken into a pudding-like consistency.
- Once the chia seed pudding has thickened, give it a good stir.
- Serve the chia seed pudding chilled, topped with your favorite fruits, nuts, or seeds.
- Enjoy your nutritious and delicious Chia Seed Breakfast Pudding!

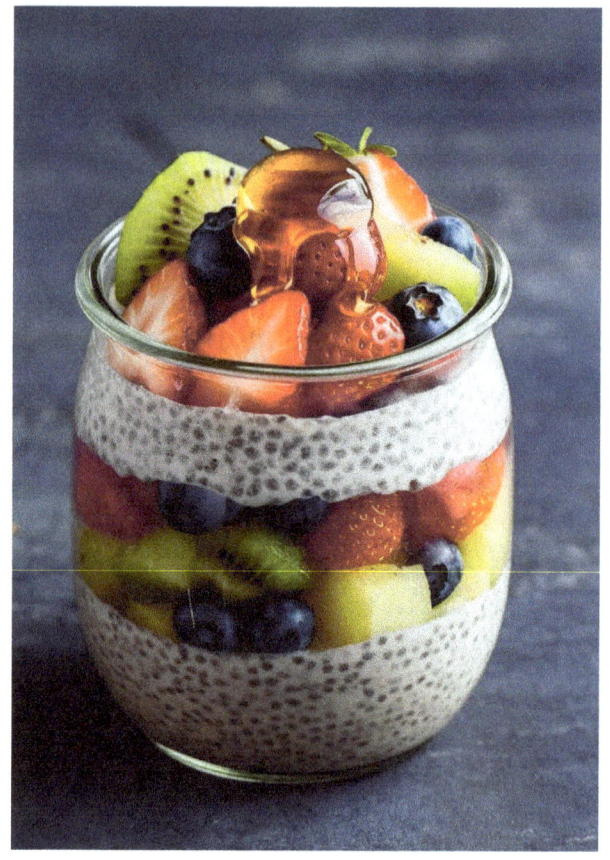

Preparation Time : 5 min
Total Time : 0 min
Servings : 1

Nutritional Info

- Calories: 220 kcal
- Protein: 6g
- Carbohydrates: 20g
- Fat: 14g
- Fiber: 10g

QUINOA AND BERRY BREAKFAST BOWL

Ingredients

- 1 cup quinoa
- 2 cups almond milk (or any milk of your choice)
- 1 tablespoon honey or maple syrup
- 1 teaspoon vanilla extract
- 1 cup mixed berries (strawberries, blueberries, raspberries)
- 1/4 cup chopped nuts (almonds, walnuts, or pecans)
- Optional toppings: sliced bananas, shredded coconut, chia seeds

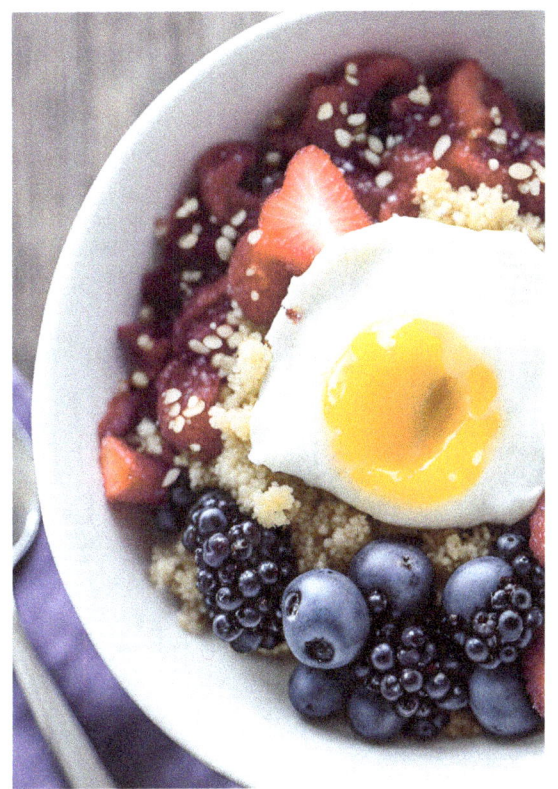

Instructions

1. Rinse quinoa under cold water using a fine mesh strainer.
2. In a medium saucepan, combine quinoa and almond milk. Bring to a boil, then reduce heat to low and simmer for 15-20 minutes, or until quinoa is cooked and liquid is absorbed.
3. Remove from heat and stir in honey or maple syrup and vanilla extract.
4. Divide the cooked quinoa into serving bowls.
5. Top each bowl with mixed berries, chopped nuts, and any other desired toppings.
6. Serve warm or chilled.

 Preparation Time : 5 min

 Total Time : 20 min

 Servings : 2

Nutritional Info

- Calories: 350 kcal
- Protein: 10g
- Carbohydrates: 55g
- Fat: 10g
- Fiber: 8g

BANANA OAT PANCAKES

Ingredients

- 1 ripe banana
- 1/2 cup rolled oats
- 2 eggs
- 1/2 teaspoon cinnamon
- 1/2 teaspoon vanilla extract
- Cooking spray or butter, for cooking
- Optional toppings: fresh berries, maple syrup, Greek yogurt

Instructions

- In a blender, combine the ripe banana, rolled oats, eggs, cinnamon, and vanilla extract. Blend until smooth.
- Heat a non-stick skillet or griddle over medium heat. Lightly coat with cooking spray or melt a small amount of butter.
- Pour the pancake batter onto the skillet, using about 1/4 cup for each pancake. Cook for 2-3 minutes, or until bubbles form on the surface.
- Flip the pancakes and cook for an additional 1-2 minutes, or until golden brown and cooked through.
- Remove the pancakes from the skillet and repeat with the remaining batter. Serve warm with your favorite toppings.

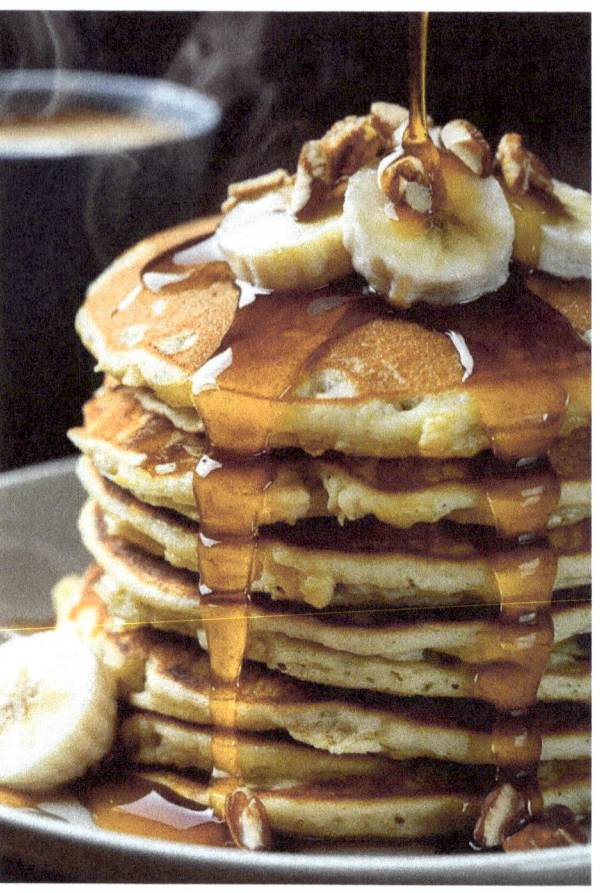

Preparation Time : 10 min

Total Time : 20 min

Servings : 2

Nutritional Info

- Calories: 250 kcal
- Protein: 10g
- Carbohydrates: 35g
- Fiber: 5g
- Sugars: 13g
- Fat: 8g

OATMEAL WITH FLAXSEEDS AND WALNUTS

Ingredients

- 1/2 cup rolled oats
- 1 cup water
- 1 tablespoon ground flaxseeds
- 2 tablespoons chopped walnuts
- Optional: honey or maple syrup for sweetness

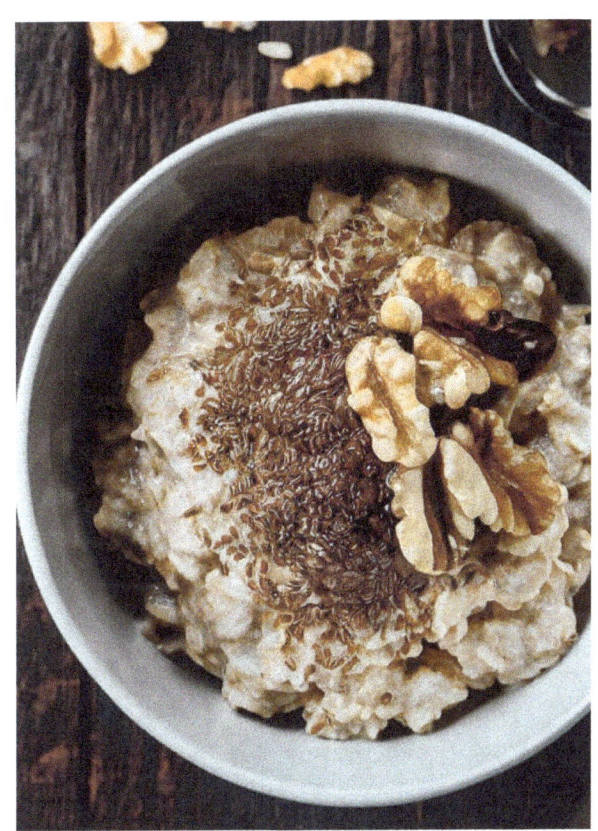

Preparation Time : 2 min

Total Time : 7 min

Servings : 1

Instructions

- In a small saucepan, bring the water to a boil.
- Stir in the rolled oats and reduce heat to medium-low.
- Cook for about 5 minutes, stirring occasionally, until the oats are tender and creamy.
- Remove from heat and stir in the ground flaxseeds.
- Transfer the oatmeal to a serving bowl and sprinkle with chopped walnuts.
- Drizzle with honey or maple syrup if desired.
- Serve hot and enjoy!

Nutritional Info

- Calories: 270 kcal
- Protein: 9g
- Carbohydrates: 38g
- Fat: 11g
- Fiber: 7g

GREEK YOGURT PARFAIT WITH FRESH BERRIES

Ingredients

- 1 cup non-fat Greek yogurt
- 1/2 cup fresh strawberries, sliced
- 1/4 cup fresh blueberries
- 1/4 cup fresh raspberries
- 1 tablespoon honey (optional)
- 1/4 cup granola (optional for added texture)

Instructions

- Wash and slice the strawberries.
- Wash the blueberries and raspberries.
- In a glass or bowl, start by adding a layer of Greek yogurt at the bottom.
- Add a layer of sliced strawberries, blueberries, and raspberries on top of the yogurt.
- Drizzle a small amount of honey over the berries if using.
- Add another layer of Greek yogurt on top of the berries.
- Repeat the layers until all ingredients are used, finishing with berries on top.
- Sprinkle granola on top for added texture and crunch, if desired.
- Serve immediately or refrigerate for up to 1 hour to allow flavors to meld.

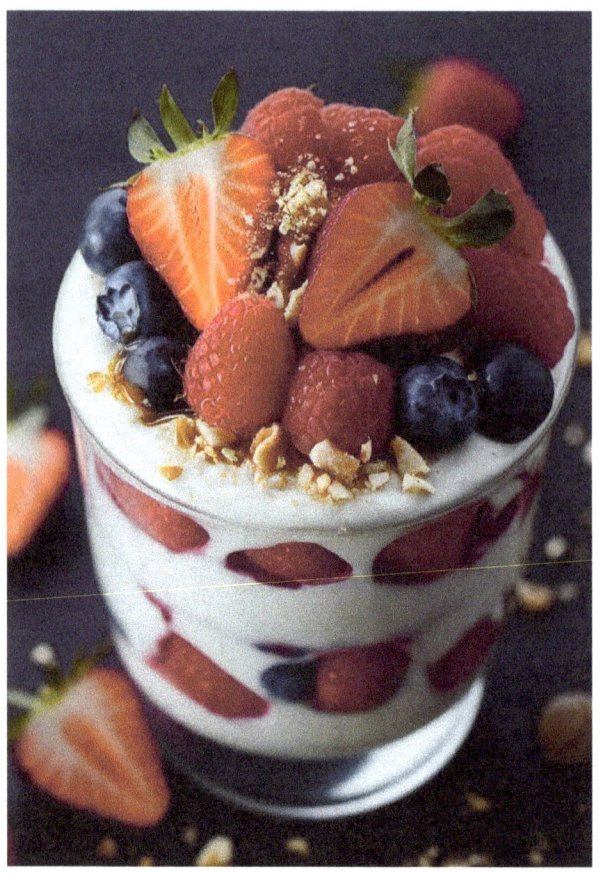

Preparation Time : 10 min

Total Time : 10 min

Servings : 1

Nutritional Info

Calories: 150
Protein: 15g
Carbohydrates: 20g
Fat: 2g
Fiber: 4g

GREEN DETOX SMOOTHIE

Ingredients

- 1 cup spinach leaves
- 1/2 cucumber, peeled and chopped
- 1/2 green apple, cored and chopped
- 1/2 lemon, juiced
- 1/2 inch fresh ginger, peeled
- 1/2 cup coconut water or plain water
- Ice cubes (optional)

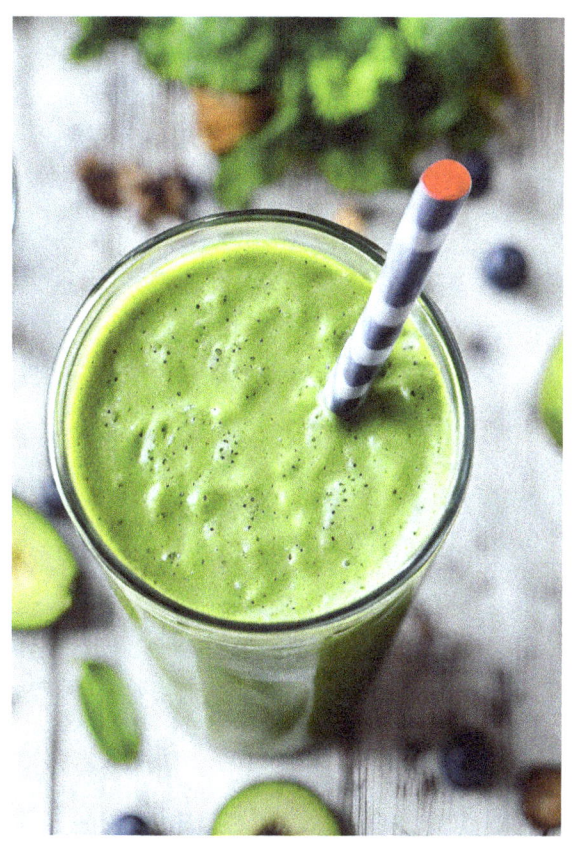

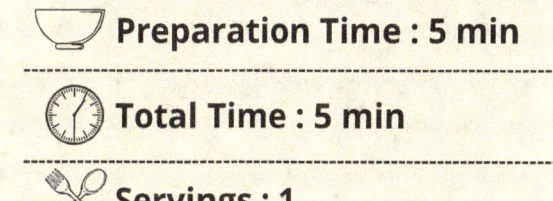

Preparation Time : 5 min

Total Time : 5 min

Servings : 1

Instructions

- Place all ingredients in a blender.
- Blend until smooth and creamy.
- Add more water if needed to reach desired consistency.
- Pour into a glass and serve immediately.

Nutritional Info

- Calories: 70
- Protein: 2g
- Carbohydrates: 16g
- Fiber: 4g
- Fat: 0.5g

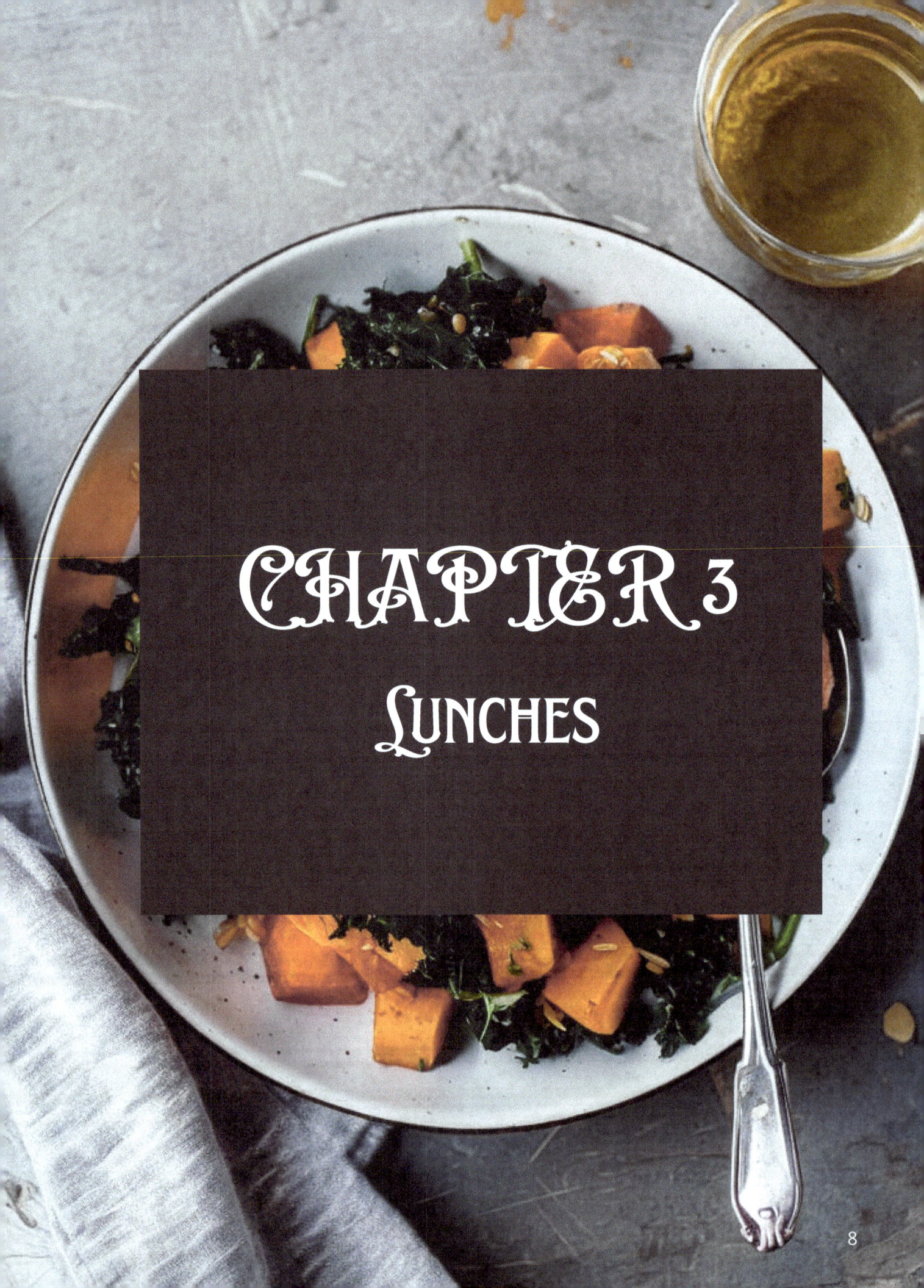

CHAPTER 3

Lunches

SPINACH AND STRAWBERRY SALAD

Ingredients

- 6 cups fresh baby spinach leaves
- 1 pint strawberries, hulled and sliced
- 1/4 cup sliced almonds
- 1/4 cup crumbled feta cheese
- Balsamic vinaigrette dressing

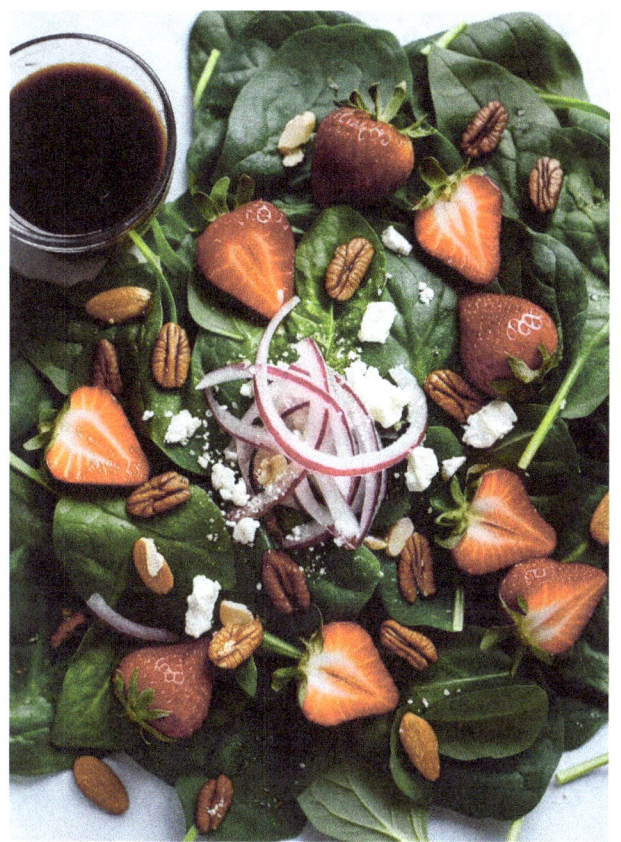

Instructions

- Wash the spinach leaves thoroughly and pat them dry with paper towels or a clean kitchen towel.
- In a large salad bowl, combine the spinach leaves, sliced strawberries, sliced almonds, and crumbled feta cheese.
- Drizzle the desired amount of balsamic vinaigrette dressing over the salad. Toss gently to coat all the ingredients evenly.
- Serve immediately as a refreshing side salad or light meal.

Preparation Time : 10 min

Total Time : 10 min

Servings : 4

Nutritional Info

- Calories: 120
- Total Fat: 7g
- Saturated Fat: 1.5g
- Cholesterol: 5mg
- Sodium: 140mg
- Dietary Fiber: 4g

GRILLED CHICKEN AND VEGETABLE SALAD

Ingredients

- 2 boneless, skinless chicken breasts
- 2 tablespoons olive oil
- 1 teaspoon garlic powder
- Salt and pepper to taste
- 4 cups mixed salad greens
- 1 bell pepper, sliced
- 1 cup cherry tomatoes, halved
- 1 small red onion, thinly sliced
- 1/4 cup balsamic vinaigrette dressing

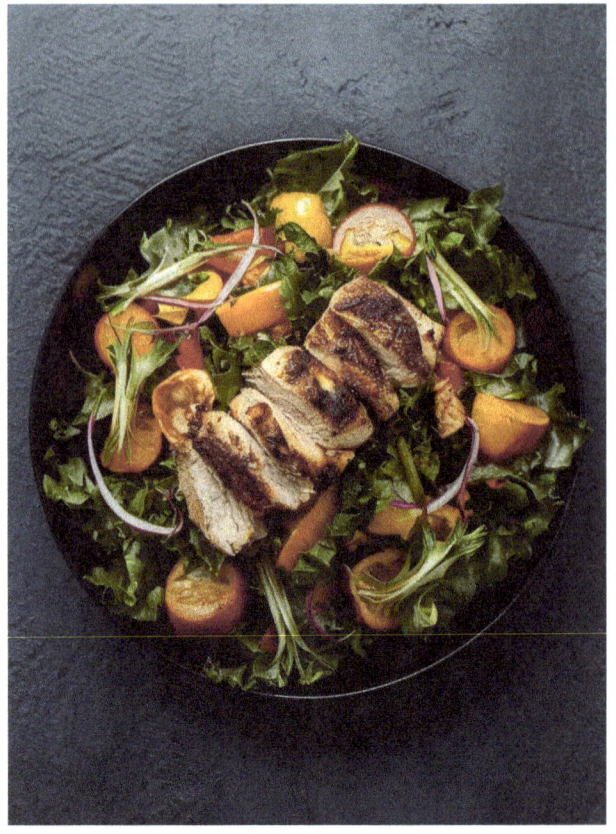

Instructions

- Preheat your grill to medium-high heat.
- In a small bowl, mix together olive oil, garlic powder, salt, and pepper. Brush this mixture onto both sides of the chicken breasts.
- Grill the chicken breasts for about 6-8 minutes per side, or until cooked through and no longer pink in the center. Remove from the grill and let them rest for a few minutes before slicing.
- While the chicken is cooking, prepare the vegetables. In a large bowl, toss together the mixed salad greens, bell pepper slices, cherry tomatoes, and red onion slices.
- Once the chicken has rested, slice it thinly.
- Arrange the grilled chicken slices on top of the salad vegetables.
- Drizzle the balsamic vinaigrette dressing over the salad.
- Serve immediately and enjoy!

 Preparation Time : 15 min

 Total Time : 30 min

 Servings : 4

Nutritional Info

- Calories: 250 kcal
- Protein: 25g
- Carbohydrates: 15g
- Fat: 10g
- Fiber: 5g

AVOCADO AND BLACK BEAN WRAP

Ingredients

- 1 can (15 oz) black beans, drained and rinsed
- 1 ripe avocado, diced
- 1 cup cherry tomatoes, halved
- 1/4 cup red onion, finely chopped
- 1/4 cup fresh cilantro, chopped
- Juice of 1 lime
- Salt and pepper to taste
- 4 whole wheat tortillas
- 1/2 cup shredded lettuce (optional)

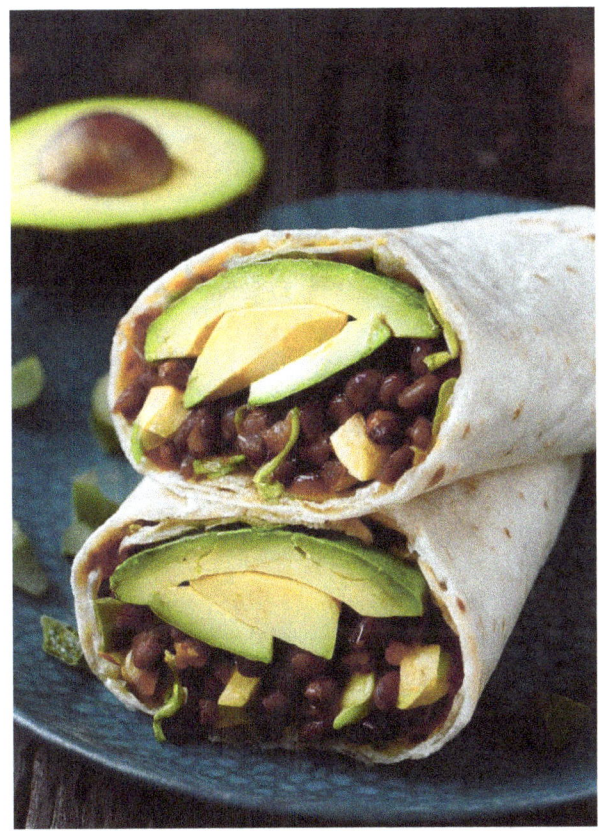

Instructions

- In a medium bowl, combine black beans, avocado, cherry tomatoes, red onion, cilantro, lime juice, salt, and pepper. Gently toss to mix all ingredients well.
- Lay the tortillas flat on a clean surface. Divide the black bean and avocado mixture evenly among the tortillas, placing it in the center of each.
- If using, sprinkle shredded lettuce over the mixture.
- Fold the sides of the tortillas over the filling, then roll them up tightly.
- Serve immediately, or wrap in foil or parchment paper to take on the go.

 Preparation Time : 10 min

 Total Time : 10 min

 Servings : 4

Nutritional Info

- Calories: 290
- Protein: 10g
- Fat: 10g
- Carbohydrates: 40g
- Fiber: 12g

ROASTED BEET AND GOAT CHEESE SALAD

Ingredients

- 4 medium beets, washed and trimmed
- 2 tablespoons olive oil
- Salt and pepper to taste
- 4 cups mixed greens (e.g., arugula, spinach, and kale)
- 1/2 cup crumbled goat cheese
- 1/4 cup chopped walnuts
- 1/4 cup balsamic vinaigrette

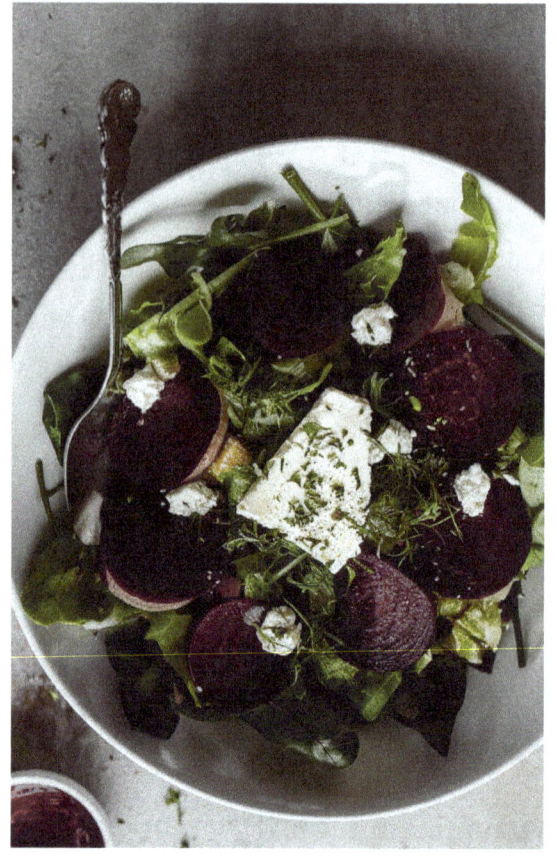

Instructions

- Preheat your oven to 400°F (200°C).
- Wrap each beet in aluminum foil and place them on a baking sheet.
- Roast for 45 minutes or until tender when pierced with a fork.
- Remove from the oven and let cool.
- Once cooled, peel the beets and cut them into wedges.
- In a large bowl, toss the mixed greens with olive oil, salt, and pepper.
- Add the roasted beet wedges, crumbled goat cheese, and chopped walnuts.
- Drizzle the balsamic vinaigrette over the salad and gently toss to combine.
- Divide the salad among four plates and serve immediately.

 Preparation Time : 15 min

 Total Time : 60 min

 Servings : 4

Nutritional Info

- Calories: 210
- Protein: 6g
- Carbohydrates: 18g
- Fat: 14g
- Fiber: 4g

SALMON AND ASPARAGUS SALAD

Ingredients

- 2 salmon fillets
- 1 bunch of asparagus, trimmed
- 2 tablespoons olive oil
- Salt and pepper to taste
- 4 cups mixed salad greens
- 1 avocado, sliced
- 1/4 cup cherry tomatoes, halved
- 2 tablespoons balsamic vinegar

Instructions

- Preheat oven to 400°F (200°C).
- Place salmon fillets on a baking sheet lined with parchment paper. Drizzle with 1 tablespoon of olive oil and season with salt and pepper. Bake for 12-15 minutes until salmon is cooked through.
- While the salmon is baking, toss asparagus spears with the remaining olive oil, salt, and pepper. Roast in the oven for 8-10 minutes until tender but still crisp.
- In a large bowl, combine mixed salad greens, avocado slices, and cherry tomatoes.
- Once the salmon and asparagus are cooked, let them cool slightly. Then, flake the salmon into chunks and add it to the salad along with the asparagus.
- Drizzle balsamic vinegar over the salad and gently toss to combine.
- Serve immediately.

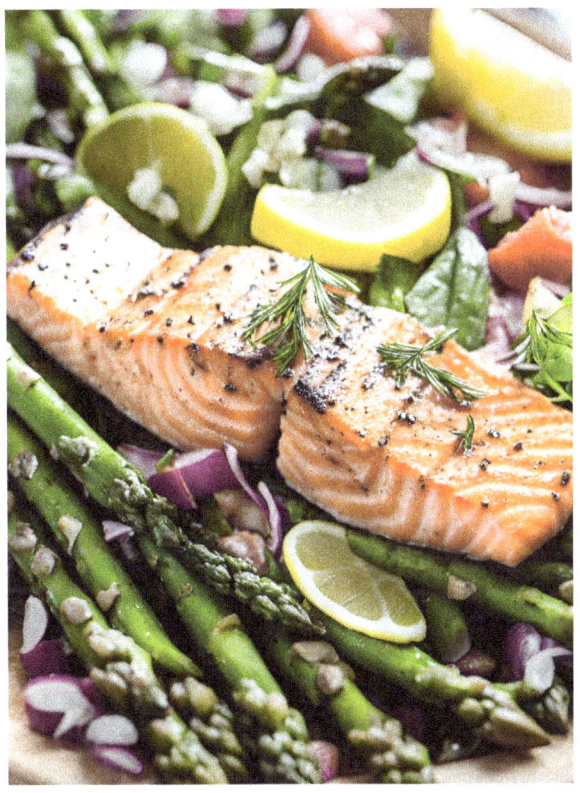

Preparation Time : 10 min

Total Time : 25 min

Servings : 2

Nutritional Info

- Calories: 450 kcal
- Protein: 28g
- Carbohydrates: 15g
- Fat: 33g
- Fiber: 9g

SWEET POTATO AND LENTIL STEW

Ingredients

- 1 tablespoon olive oil
- 1 onion, chopped
- 2 cloves garlic, minced
- 2 medium sweet potatoes, peeled and diced
- 1 cup dried green lentils, rinsed
- 4 cups vegetable broth
- 1 can (14 ounces) diced tomatoes
- 1 teaspoon ground cumin
- 1 teaspoon ground coriander
- Salt and pepper to taste

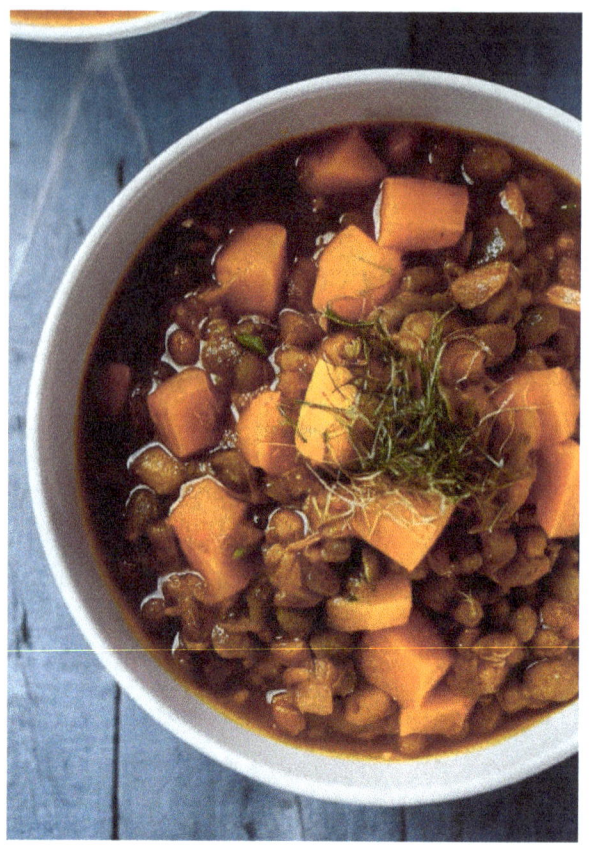

Instructions

- In a large pot or Dutch oven, heat the olive oil over medium heat.
- Add the chopped onion and minced garlic. Sauté until the onion is translucent, about 3-4 minutes.
- Add the diced sweet potatoes and rinsed lentils to the pot.
- Pour in the vegetable broth and diced tomatoes. Stir to combine.
- Season the stew with ground cumin, ground coriander, salt, and pepper.
- Bring the stew to a simmer, then reduce the heat to low. Cover and cook for 25-30 minutes, or until the sweet potatoes and lentils are tender.
- Taste and adjust seasoning if needed.
- Serve the stew hot, garnished with fresh cilantro or parsley if desired.

 Preparation Time : 10 min

 Total Time : 40 min

 Servings : 4

Nutritional Info

- Calories: 315 kcal
- Protein: 13g
- Carbohydrates: 58g
- Fat: 4g
- Fiber: 15g

TOFU AND BROCCOLI STIR-FRY

Ingredients

- 1 block firm tofu, drained and cubed
- 2 cups broccoli florets
- 2 tablespoons soy sauce (or tamari for gluten-free)
- 1 tablespoon sesame oil
- 2 cloves garlic, minced
- 1 tablespoon grated ginger
- 2 tablespoons olive oil (for cooking)

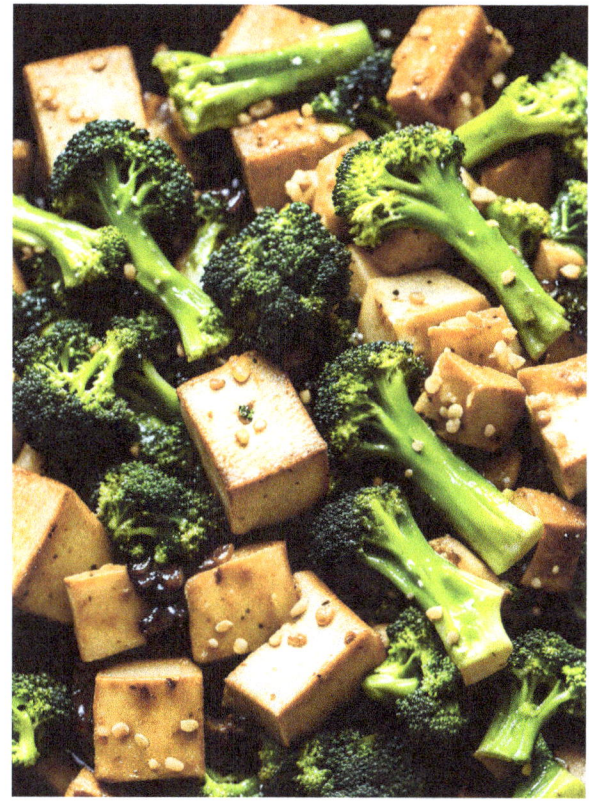

Instructions

- Heat olive oil in a large skillet or wok over medium-high heat.
- Add cubed tofu to the skillet and cook until golden brown on all sides, about 5-7 minutes. Remove tofu from skillet and set aside.
- In the same skillet, add broccoli florets and cook for 3-4 minutes until they are bright green and slightly tender.
- Add minced garlic and grated ginger to the skillet, stirring constantly for about 1 minute until fragrant.
- Return the cooked tofu to the skillet and pour soy sauce and sesame oil over the tofu and broccoli mixture. Stir well to coat everything evenly.
- Cook for an additional 2-3 minutes until the sauce has thickened slightly and everything is heated through.
- Remove from heat and garnish with sesame seeds and sliced green onions if desired.
- Serve hot over cooked rice or quinoa.

 Preparation Time : 10min

 Total Time : 20 min

 Servings : 2

Nutritional Info

- Calories: 250 kcal
- Protein: 15g
- Carbohydrates: 10g
- Fat: 18g
- Fiber: 5g

SPICY TUNA AND AVOCADO BOWL

Ingredients

- 1 can (5 oz) of tuna in water, drained
- 1 ripe avocado, diced
- 1 cup cooked brown rice (optional, adjust points if included)
- 1 cup mixed greens
- 1/2 cup shredded carrots
- 1/2 cup sliced cucumber
- 1/4 cup chopped green onions
- 1 tbsp soy sauce (low sodium)
- 1 tsp sesame oil
- 1 tsp Sriracha (adjust to taste)
- 1 tbsp lime juice
- 1 tbsp sesame seeds

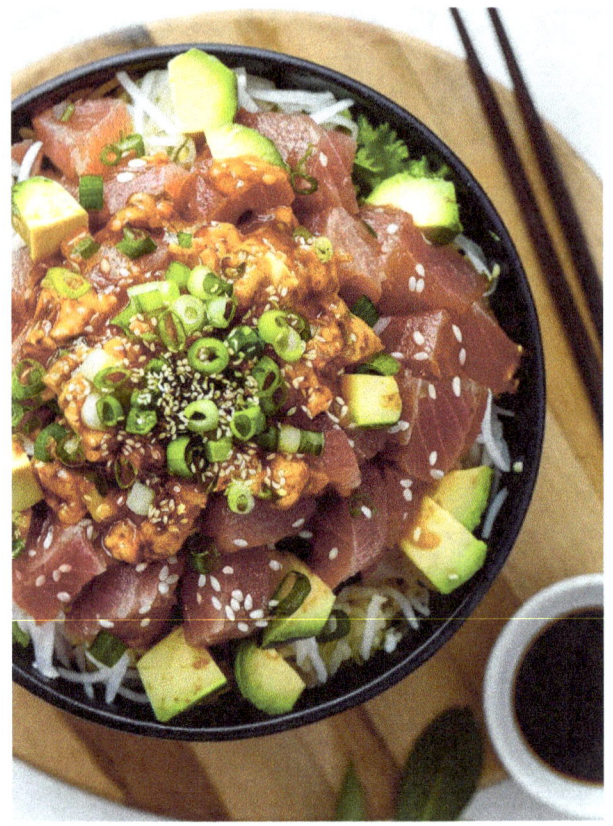

Instructions

- Prepare the Ingredients: Drain the tuna and place it in a medium bowl. Dice the avocado and set aside. Cook the brown rice if using.
- Make the Dressing: In a small bowl, whisk together the soy sauce, sesame oil, Sriracha, and lime juice.
- Combine Ingredients: In the bowl with the tuna, add the mixed greens, shredded carrots, sliced cucumber, chopped green onions, and diced avocado. Pour the dressing over the mixture.
- Mix Well: Gently toss all the ingredients together until evenly coated with the dressing.
- Serve: Divide the mixture into bowls, sprinkle with sesame seeds, and season with salt and pepper to taste. Serve immediately.
- Optional: Serve over a bed of cooked brown rice for a heartier meal.

Preparation Time : 10 min

Total Time : 10 min

Servings : 1

Nutritional Info

- Calories: 320 (without brown rice)
- Protein: 20g
- Carbohydrates: 14g
- Fat: 22g
- Fiber: 8g

CHICKEN CAESAR SALAD

Ingredients

- 2 boneless, skinless chicken breasts
- 1 tablespoon olive oil
- 1 teaspoon garlic powder
- Salt and pepper to taste
- 1 large head of romaine lettuce, chopped
- 1/2 cup cherry tomatoes, halved
- 1/4 cup grated Parmesan cheese
- 1/2 cup croutons (optional)
- Lemon wedges for garnish

Instructions

- Preheat your oven to 375°F (190°C).
- Rub the chicken breasts with olive oil, garlic powder, salt, and pepper.
- Place the chicken breasts on a baking sheet and bake for 20 minutes, or until the internal temperature reaches 165°F (74°C).
- Allow the chicken to rest for 5 minutes before slicing.
- While the chicken is baking, chop the romaine lettuce and place it in a large salad bowl.
- Add the halved cherry tomatoes and grated Parmesan cheese to the bowl.
- If using croutons, add them to the salad as well.
- Once the chicken has rested, slice it into thin strips.
- Arrange the sliced chicken on top of the salad.
- Serve the salad with lemon wedges on the side for squeezing over the top.
- Divide the salad into four servings.
- Enjoy your Chicken Caesar Salad without dressing, optionally squeezing fresh lemon juice over the top for extra flavor.

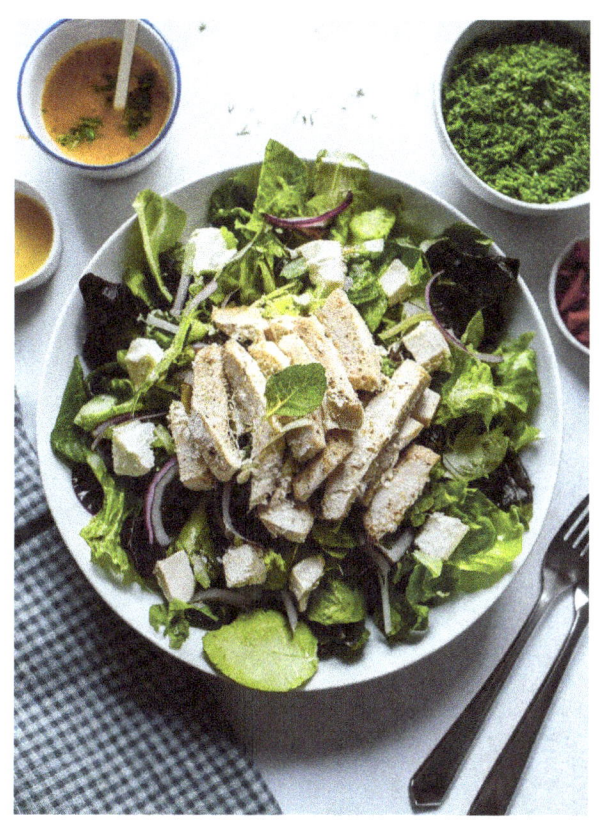

 Preparation Time : 15 min

 Total Time : 35 min

 Servings : 4

Nutritional Info

- Calories: 220
- Protein: 30g
- Carbohydrates: 8g
- Fat: 8g
- Fiber: 2g

MEDITERRANEAN CHICKPEA BOWL

Ingredients

- 1 can (15 oz) chickpeas, drained and rinsed
- 1 cup cherry tomatoes, halved
- 1 cucumber, diced
- 1/2 red onion, thinly sliced
- 1/4 cup Kalamata olives, pitted and sliced
- 2 tablespoons extra virgin olive oil
- 1 tablespoon lemon juice
- 1 teaspoon dried oregano
- Salt and pepper to taste

Instructions

- In a large bowl, combine the chickpeas, cherry tomatoes, cucumber, red onion, and Kalamata olives.
- In a small bowl, whisk together the extra virgin olive oil, lemon juice, dried oregano, salt, and pepper.
- Pour the dressing over the chickpea mixture and toss until well combined.
- Divide the chickpea mixture into serving bowls.
- Top with crumbled feta cheese and fresh parsley if desired.
- Serve immediately and enjoy!

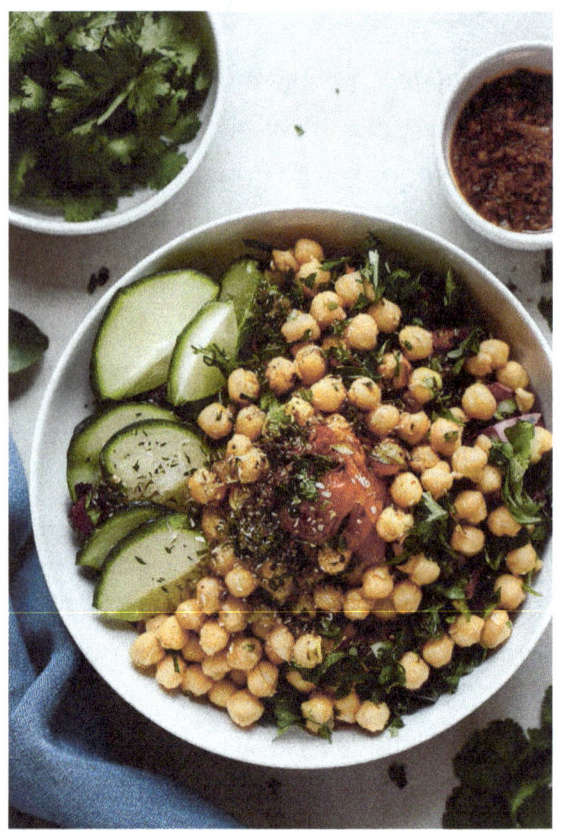

 Preparation Time : 10 min

 Total Time : 10 min

 Servings : 2

Nutritional Info

- Calories: 320 kcal
- Total Fat: 18g
- Saturated Fat: 2.5g
- Trans Fat: 0g
- Cholesterol: 0mg

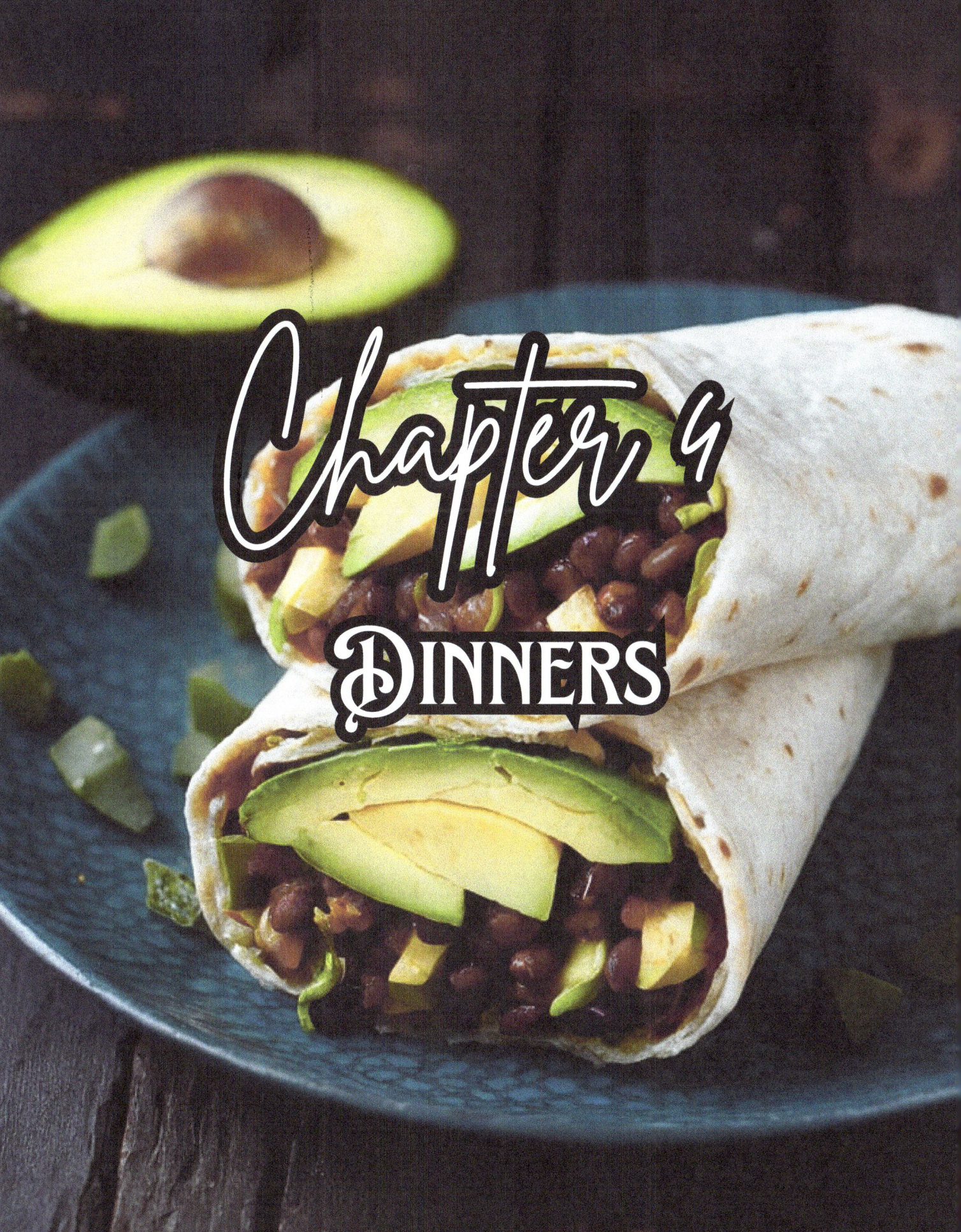

Chapter 4
Dinners

BAKED SALMON WITH LEMON AND DILL

Ingredients

- 4 salmon fillets
- 2 tablespoons olive oil
- 2 tablespoons fresh lemon juice
- 2 cloves garlic, minced
- 1 tablespoon fresh dill, chopped
- Salt and pepper, to taste
- Lemon slices, for garnish

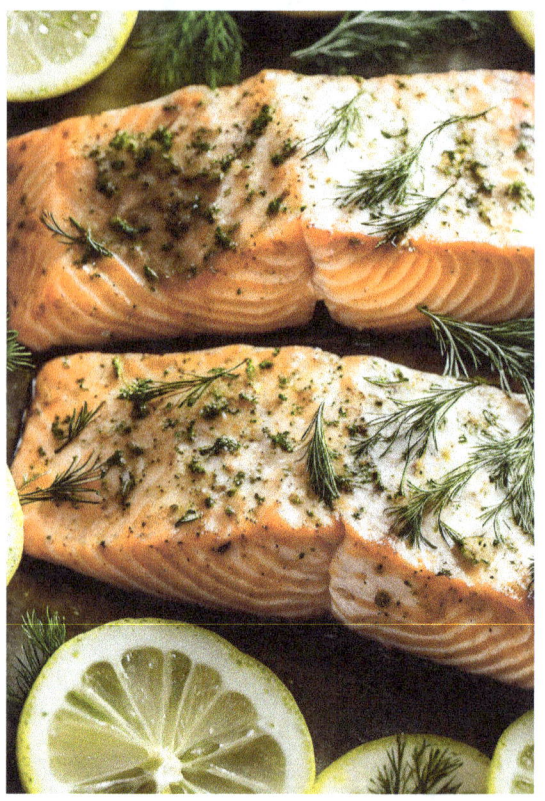

Instructions

- Preheat your oven to 375°F (190°C). Line a baking sheet with parchment paper or lightly grease it with olive oil.
- In a small bowl, mix together the olive oil, lemon juice, minced garlic, chopped dill, salt, and pepper.
- Place the salmon fillets on the prepared baking sheet. Brush each fillet with the lemon-dill mixture, coating them evenly.
- Place a lemon slice on top of each salmon fillet for added flavor.
- Bake the salmon in the preheated oven for 12-15 minutes, or until the salmon is cooked through and flakes easily with a fork.
- Once done, remove the salmon from the oven and garnish with fresh dill sprigs.
- Serve the baked salmon hot with your favorite side dishes.

Preparation Time : 10 min

Total Time : 20 min

Servings : 4

Nutritional Info

- Calories: 280 kcal
- Protein: 25g
- Fat: 18g
- Carbohydrates: 2g
- Fiber: 0.5g

QUINOA AND VEGETABLE STUFFED PEPPERS

Ingredients

- 4 large bell peppers, any color
- 1 cup quinoa, rinsed
- 2 cups vegetable broth
- 1 tablespoon olive oil
- 1 onion, diced
- 2 cloves garlic, minced
- 1 zucchini, diced
- 1 carrot, diced
- 1 cup diced tomatoes
- 1 teaspoon dried oregano
- Salt and pepper to taste

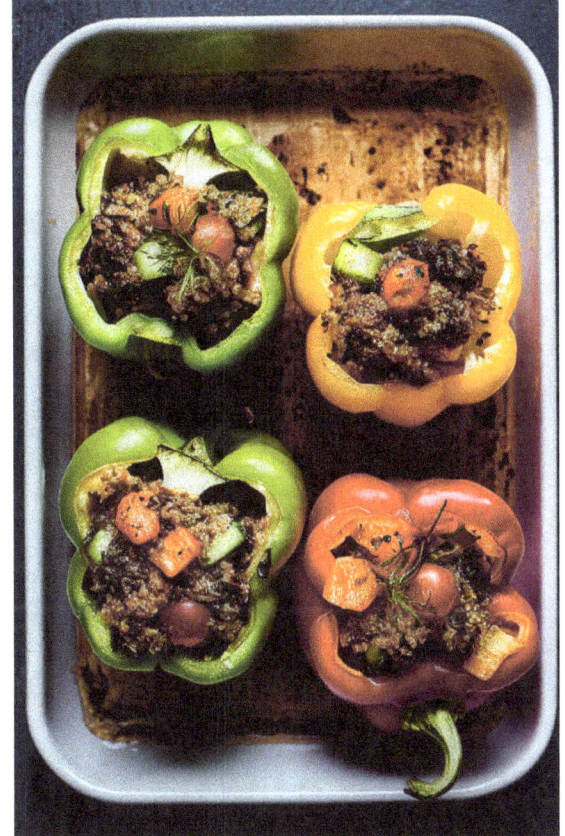

Instructions

- Preheat oven to 375°F (190°C).
- Cook quinoa: In a saucepan, combine quinoa and vegetable broth. Bring to a boil, then simmer covered for 15 minutes until cooked.
- Prepare vegetables: Heat olive oil in a skillet. Add onion and garlic, cook until softened (about 5 mins). Then add zucchini and carrot, cook for another 5 mins until tender.
- Mix: Stir in diced tomatoes, oregano, cooked quinoa, salt, and pepper. Cook for 2-3 more minutes.
- Prepare peppers: Cut the tops off the bell peppers, remove seeds and membranes. Place in a baking dish.
- Fill peppers: Spoon quinoa and vegetable mixture into each pepper.
- Optional: Sprinkle shredded mozzarella cheese on top.
- Bake: Cover dish with foil, bake for 25-30 mins until peppers are tender.
- Serve hot and enjoy!

 Preparation Time : 20 min

 Total Time : 1 hour

Servings : 4

Nutritional Info

- Calories: 295 kcal
- Total Fat: 7g
- Saturated Fat: 1g
- Cholesterol: 0mg
- Sodium: 460mg

TURMERIC CHICKEN AND RICE

Ingredients

- 1 lb boneless, skinless chicken breasts, cut into bite-sized pieces
- 2 cups white or brown rice
- 1 tablespoon olive oil
- 1 onion, chopped
- 3 cloves garlic, minced
- 1 tablespoon ground turmeric
- 1 teaspoon ground cumin
- 1 teaspoon ground coriander
- Salt and pepper to taste
- 3 cups chicken broth
- 1 cup frozen peas

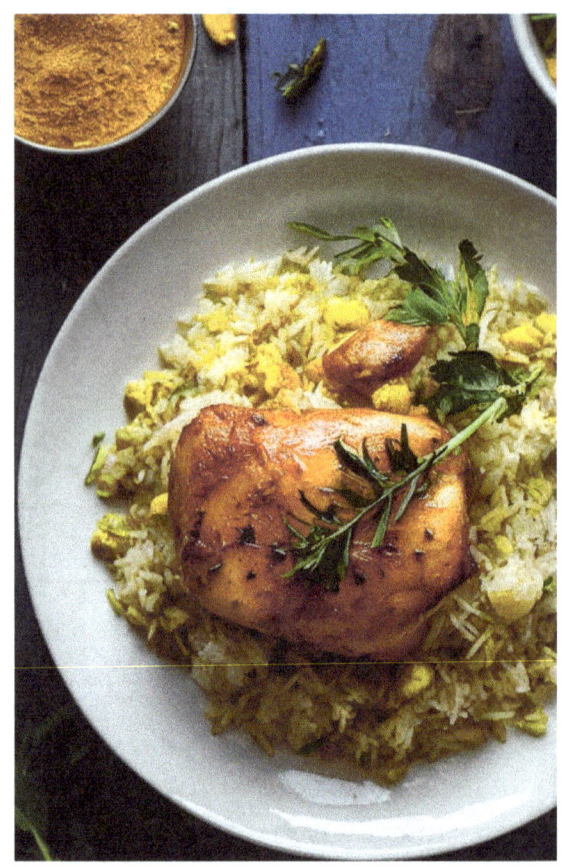

Instructions

- Heat olive oil in a large skillet over medium heat. Add chopped onion and minced garlic, sauté until softened.
- Add chicken pieces to the skillet, cook until browned on all sides.
- Stir in ground turmeric, cumin, and coriander, coating the chicken evenly.
- Add rice to the skillet, stirring to combine with the chicken and spices.
- Pour chicken broth into the skillet, bring to a boil.
- Reduce heat to low, cover, and simmer for 20-25 minutes or until rice is cooked and liquid is absorbed.
- Stir in frozen peas, cover, and cook for an additional 5 minutes until peas are heated through.
- Garnish with chopped cilantro before serving.

 Preparation Time : 10 min

 Total Time : 35 min

 Servings : 4

Nutritional Info

- Calories: 400 kcal
- Protein: 30g
- Carbohydrates: 45g
- Fat: 10g
- Fiber: 4g

SWEET POTATO AND BLACK BEAN ENCHILADAS

Ingredients

- 2 medium sweet potatoes, peeled and diced
- 1 can (15 oz) black beans, drained and rinsed
- 1 cup corn kernels (fresh or frozen)
- 1 bell pepper, diced
- 1 small onion, diced
- 2 cloves garlic, minced
- 1 teaspoon ground cumin
- 1 teaspoon chili powder
- Salt and pepper, to taste
- 8 small corn tortillas
- 1 cup enchilada sauce
- 1 cup shredded cheese

Instructions

- Preheat oven to 375°F (190°C). Grease a baking dish.
- In a skillet over medium heat, cook sweet potatoes until soft, about 5-7 minutes.
- Add onion, bell pepper, and garlic. Cook until tender, about 5 minutes.
- Stir in black beans, corn, cumin, chili powder, salt, and pepper. Cook for 2-3 minutes.
- Warm tortillas in the microwave for 30 seconds.
- Spoon filling onto each tortilla. Roll up and place seam-side down in the baking dish.
- Pour enchilada sauce over the top. Sprinkle cheese evenly.
- Cover with foil and bake for 20 minutes.
- Remove foil and bake for 5-10 more minutes, until cheese melts.
- Garnish with cilantro if desired before serving.

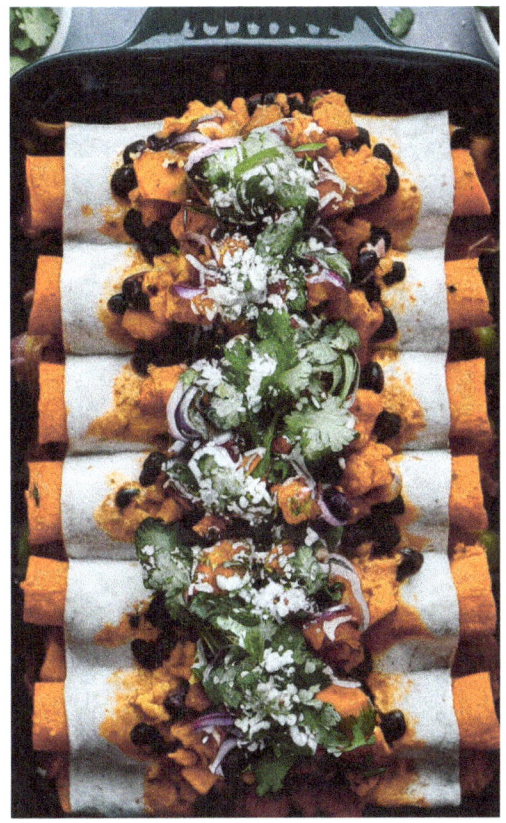

Preparation Time : 15 min

Total Time : 35 min

Servings : 4

Nutritional Info

- Calories: 380
- Total Fat: 10g
- Saturated Fat: 5g
- Cholesterol: 20mg
- Sodium: 680mg
- Total Carbohydrates: 59g

ZUCCHINI NOODLES WITH PESTO

Ingredients

- 4 medium zucchinis, spiralized
- 1 cup fresh basil leaves
- 1/4 cup pine nuts
- 2 cloves garlic
- 1/4 cup grated Parmesan cheese
- 1/4 cup olive oil
- Salt and pepper to taste

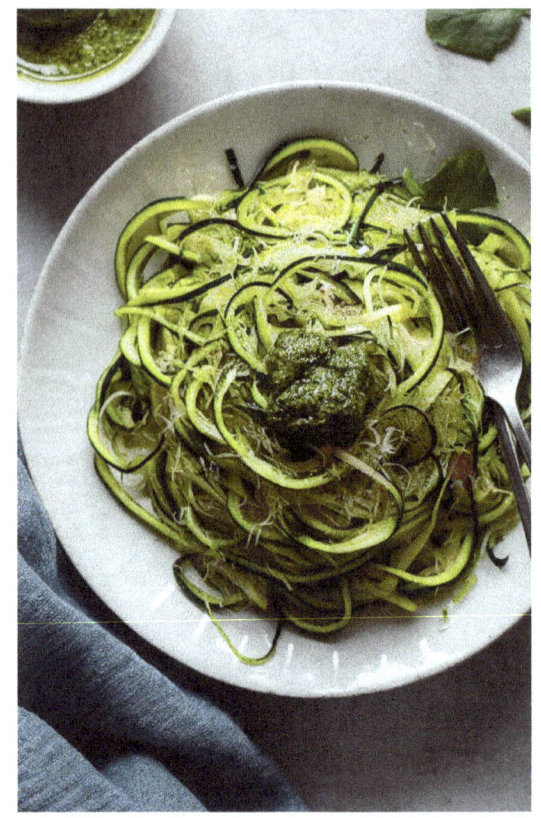

Instructions

- In a food processor, combine basil leaves, pine nuts, garlic, and Parmesan cheese. Pulse until finely chopped.
- With the processor running, slowly drizzle in the olive oil until the mixture forms a smooth paste. Season with salt and pepper to taste.
- In a large skillet over medium heat, add the spiralized zucchini noodles. Cook for 2-3 minutes until slightly softened but still crisp.
- Add the pesto sauce to the skillet with the zucchini noodles and toss until well coated.
- Serve immediately, garnished with sliced cherry tomatoes if desired.

Preparation Time : 10 min
Total Time : 15 min
Servings : 4

Nutritional Info

- Calories: 180 kcal
- Protein: 5g
- Fat: 16g
- Carbohydrates: 7g
- Fiber: 2g

HERB-ROASTED CHICKEN AND VEGETABLES

Ingredients

- 4 bone-in, skin-on chicken thighs
- 2 cups baby potatoes, halved
- 2 cups carrots, peeled and sliced into sticks
- 1 cup Brussels sprouts, halved
- 2 tablespoons olive oil
- 2 cloves garlic, minced
- 1 teaspoon dried thyme
- 1 teaspoon dried rosemary
- 1 teaspoon dried oregano
- Salt and pepper to taste

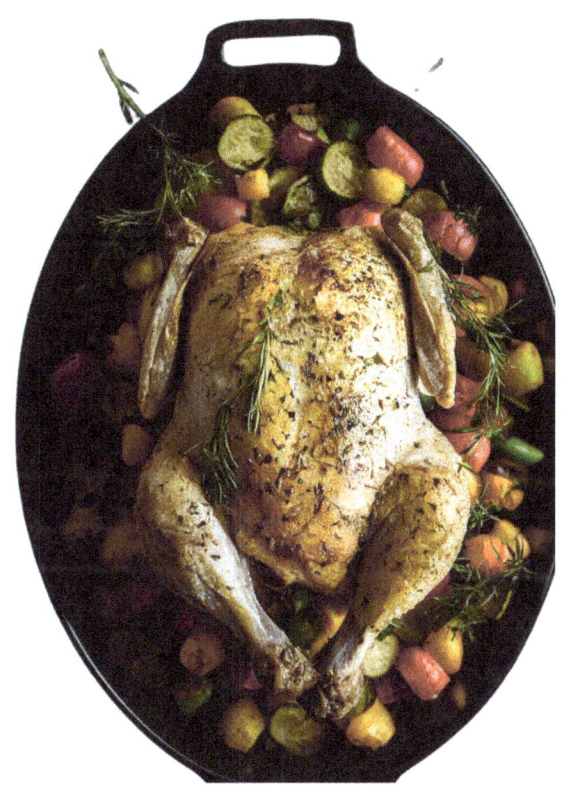

Instructions

- Preheat your oven to 400°F (200°C).
- In a large mixing bowl, combine the chicken thighs, potatoes, carrots, Brussels sprouts, olive oil, minced garlic, dried thyme, dried rosemary, dried oregano, salt, and pepper. Toss until everything is evenly coated.
- Transfer the chicken and vegetable mixture to a baking sheet lined with parchment paper or aluminum foil, arranging everything in a single layer.
- Roast in the preheated oven for 35-40 minutes or until the chicken is cooked through and the vegetables are tender and golden brown.
- Serve hot, garnished with fresh herbs if desired.

Preparation Time : 15 min

Total Time : 55 min

Servings : 4

Nutritional Info

- Calories: 380 kcal
- Total Fat: 20g
- Saturated Fat: 5g
- Trans Fat: 0g
- Cholesterol: 120mg
- Sodium: 210mg

GINGER-GARLIC SHRIMP STIR-FRY

Ingredients

- 1 lb shrimp, peeled and deveined
- 2 tablespoons olive oil
- 3 cloves garlic, minced
- 1 tablespoon fresh ginger, minced
- 1 red bell pepper, thinly sliced
- 1 yellow bell pepper, thinly sliced
- 1 cup snow peas
- 1/4 cup low-sodium soy sauce
- 2 tablespoons honey
- 2 green onions, chopped

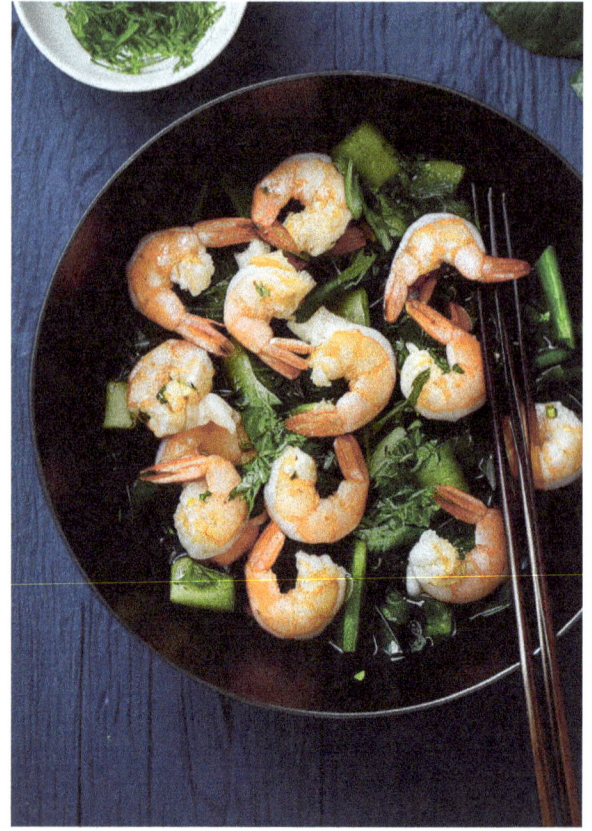

Instructions

- In a large pan, heat olive oil over medium-high heat.
- Add garlic and ginger, sauté for 1-2 minutes until fragrant.
- Add shrimp and cook for 3-4 minutes until pink and cooked through.
- Stir in bell peppers and snow peas, cook for an additional 2-3 minutes.
- In a small bowl, mix soy sauce and honey. Pour over the shrimp and vegetables, stirring to combine.
- Cook for another 1-2 minutes, until the sauce has thickened slightly.
- Remove from heat and sprinkle with chopped green onions.
- Serve over cooked rice.

Preparation Time : 15 min

Total Time : 25 min

Servings : 4

Nutritional Info

- Calories: 280
- Protein: 25g
- Fat: 10g
- Carbohydrates: 20g
- Fiber: 3g

LENTIL AND SPINACH CURRY

Ingredients

- 1 cup dried lentils
- 2 cups fresh spinach, chopped
- 1 onion, finely chopped
- 2 cloves garlic, minced
- 1 tablespoon curry powder
- 1 teaspoon ground cumin
- 1 teaspoon ground coriander
- 1 can (14 ounces) diced tomatoes
- 1 can (14 ounces) coconut milk
- Salt and pepper, to taste

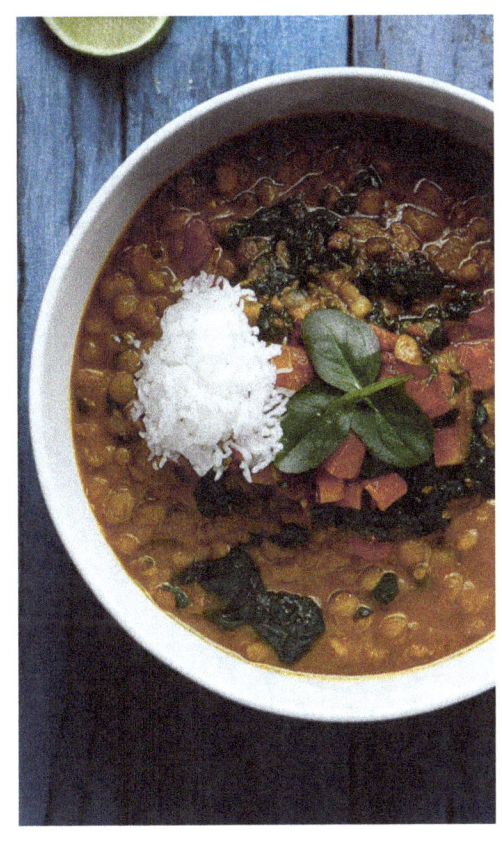

Instructions

- Rinse the lentils under cold water until the water runs clear. Drain well.
- In a large pot or skillet, heat some oil over medium heat. Add the chopped onion and minced garlic, and sauté until softened and fragrant, about 3-4 minutes.
- Stir in the curry powder, ground cumin, and ground coriander. Cook for another minute until the spices are toasted and fragrant.
- Add the rinsed lentils, diced tomatoes (with their juices), and coconut milk to the pot. Stir to combine.
- Bring the mixture to a boil, then reduce the heat to low. Cover and simmer for about 20-25 minutes, or until the lentils are tender and cooked through.
- Stir in the chopped spinach and cook for an additional 2-3 minutes, until the spinach is wilted.
- Season with salt and pepper to taste.
- Serve the lentil and spinach curry hot over cooked rice. Garnish with fresh cilantro.

 Preparation Time : 10 min

 Total Time : 35 min

 Servings : 4

Nutritional Info

- Calories: 320 kcal
- Protein: 15g
- Carbohydrates: 40g
- Fat: 12g
- Fiber: 14g

ROASTED CAULIFLOWER STEAKS

Ingredients

- 1 large head of cauliflower
- 2-3 tablespoons olive oil
- Salt and pepper to taste
- Optional: your favorite seasoning blend (such as garlic powder, smoked paprika, or cumin)

Instructions

- Preheat your oven to 425°F (220°C).
- Remove the outer leaves of the cauliflower and trim the stem end to create a flat base.
- Place the cauliflower head on a cutting board and slice it vertically into 1-inch thick slices, creating "steaks." You should get 2-3 steaks from one head of cauliflower.
- Place the cauliflower steaks on a baking sheet lined with parchment paper or aluminum foil.
- Drizzle olive oil over the cauliflower steaks and use your hands to rub it evenly on both sides.
- Season the cauliflower steaks with salt, pepper, and any optional seasoning blend of your choice.
- Roast in the preheated oven for 25-30 minutes, flipping halfway through, until the cauliflower is tender and golden brown on the edges.

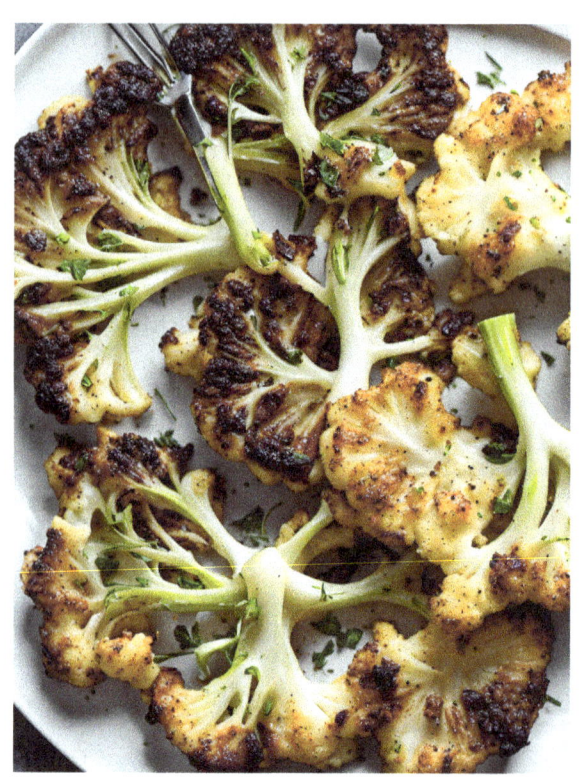

 Preparation Time : 10 min

 Total Time : 35 min

 Servings : 2-3

Nutritional Info

- Calories: 120 kcal
- Protein: 5g
- Fat: 9g
- Carbohydrates: 10g
- Fiber: 5g

BAKED COD WITH TOMATO AND OLIVE RELISH

Ingredients

- 4 cod fillets (about 6 oz each)
- 1 cup cherry tomatoes, halved
- 1/4 cup Kalamata olives, chopped
- 2 tablespoons olive oil
- 2 cloves garlic, minced
- 1 tablespoon fresh lemon juice
- Salt and pepper to taste
- Fresh parsley, chopped (for garnish)

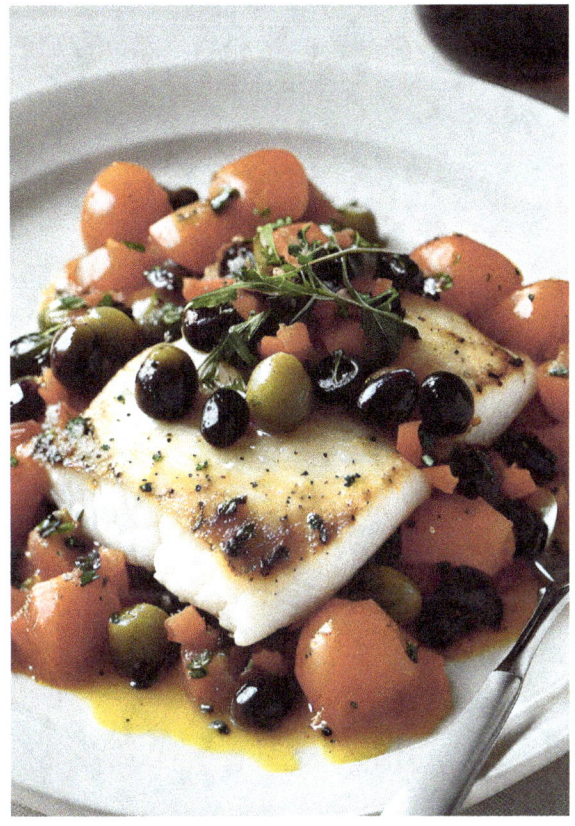

Instructions

- Preheat the oven to 400°F (200°C).
- Place the cod fillets on a baking dish lined with parchment paper.
- In a small bowl, mix the cherry tomatoes, olives, olive oil, garlic, lemon juice, salt, and pepper.
- Spoon the tomato and olive mixture over the cod fillets.
- Bake for 15-20 minutes, or until the fish is cooked through and flakes easily with a fork.
- Garnish with fresh parsley before serving.

Preparation Time : 10 min
Total Time : 25 min
Servings : 4

Nutritional Info

- Calories: 300
- Protein: 30g
- Fat: 14g
- Carbohydrates: 8g
- Fiber: 2g

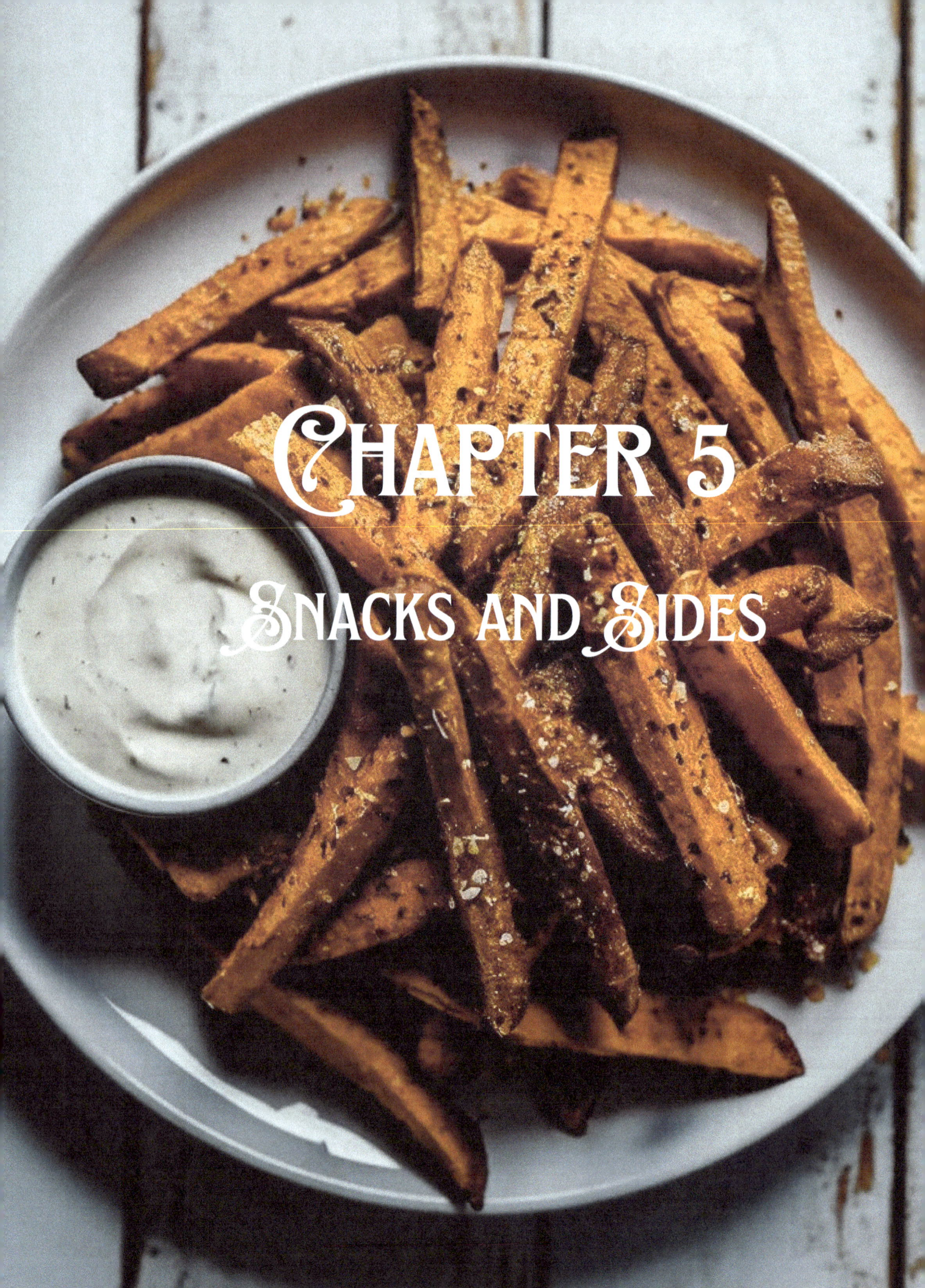

Chapter 5

Snacks and Sides

EDAMAME WITH SEA SALT

Ingredients

- 2 cups frozen edamame in pods
- 1 tablespoon sea salt (or to taste)
- Water for boiling

Instructions

- Fill a large pot with water and bring it to a boil over high heat.
- Once the water is boiling, add the frozen edamame pods to the pot.
- Boil for 5 minutes, or until the edamame pods are tender and easily open when squeezed.
- Drain the edamame in a colander and rinse under cold water to stop the cooking process.
- Transfer the edamame to a bowl and sprinkle with sea salt. Toss to evenly coat the pods with the salt.
- Serve immediately as a snack or appetizer.
- To eat, simply squeeze the edamame beans out of the pods and discard the pods.

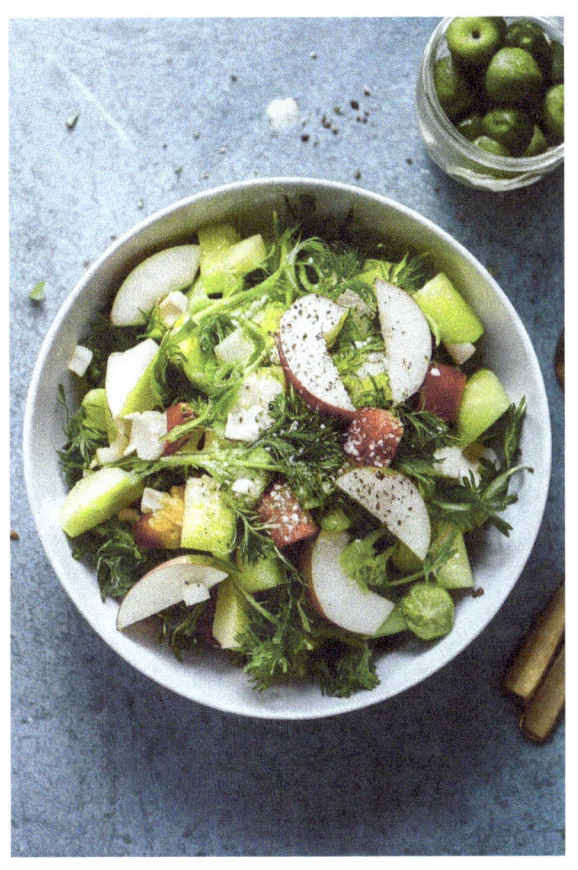

 Preparation Time : 5 min

 Total Time : 15 min

 Servings : 4

Nutritional Info

- Calories: 120
- Protein: 12g
- Carbohydrates: 10g
- Fat: 5g
- Fiber: 4g
- Sodium: 150mg

SPICED SWEET POTATO FRIES

Ingredients

- 2 large sweet potatoes
- 1 teaspoon paprika
- 1/2 teaspoon garlic powder
- 1/2 teaspoon onion powder
- 1/2 teaspoon ground cumin
- 1/4 teaspoon cayenne pepper (optional)
- Salt and pepper to taste

Instructions

- Preheat Oven: Preheat oven to 425°F (220°C). Line a baking sheet with parchment paper or spray with cooking spray.
- Cut Sweet Potatoes: Peel and cut sweet potatoes into thin fries.
- Season: Mix paprika, garlic powder, onion powder, cumin, cayenne pepper (if using), salt, and pepper in a large bowl. Add sweet potatoes and toss to coat.
- Bake: Spread fries on the baking sheet in a single layer. Bake for 20-25 minutes, turning halfway through, until golden and crispy.
- Serve: Let cool slightly and enjoy!

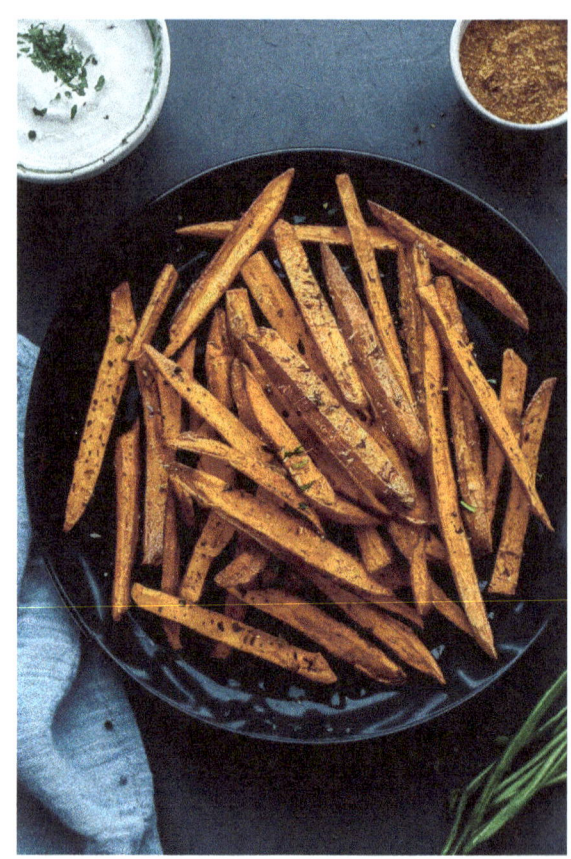

Preparation Time : 10 min

Total Time : 35 min

Servings : 4

Nutritional Info

- Calories: 120
- Protein: 2g
- Carbohydrates: 27g
- Fiber: 4g
- Fat: 0.5g

GUACAMOLE WITH VEGGIE STICKS

Ingredients

- 2 ripe avocados
- 1 small tomato, diced
- 1/4 cup red onion, finely chopped
- 1 jalapeño pepper, seeded and minced (optional for spice)
- 2 tablespoons fresh cilantro, chopped
- 1 tablespoon lime juice
- Salt and pepper to taste

Instructions

- Cut the avocados in half, remove the pits, and scoop the flesh into a mixing bowl.
- Mash the avocados with a fork until smooth or until your desired consistency is reached.
- Add the diced tomato, chopped red onion, minced jalapeño pepper (if using), chopped cilantro, and lime juice to the bowl with the mashed avocado.
- Season with salt and pepper to taste.
- Stir all the ingredients until well combined.
- Taste and adjust seasoning if necessary.
- Transfer the guacamole to a serving bowl and garnish with additional cilantro if desired.
- Serve the guacamole with assorted vegetable sticks for dipping.

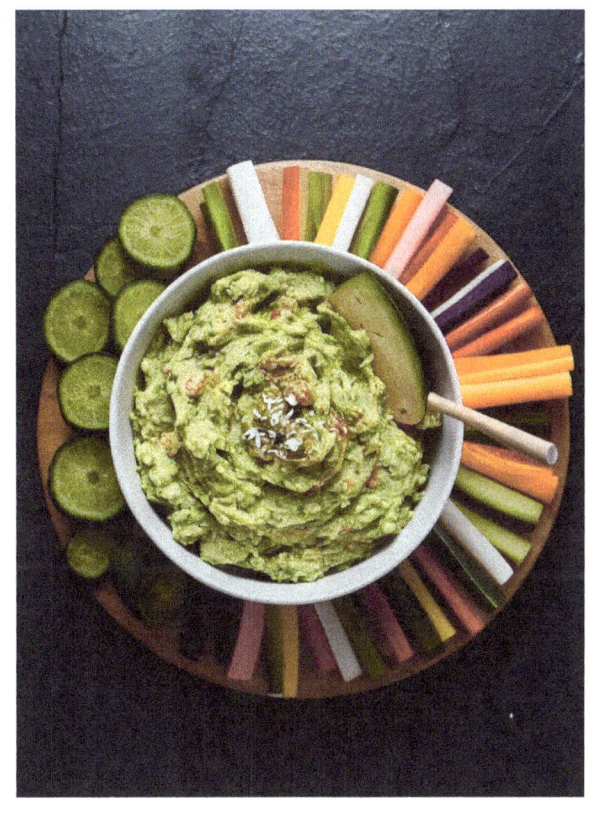

 Preparation Time : 10 min

 Total Time : 10 min

 Servings : 4

Nutritional Info

- Calories: 120
- Total Fat: 10g
- Saturated Fat: 1.5g
- Sodium: 250mg
- Total Carbohydrates: 8g
- Dietary Fiber: 6g

ROASTED CHICKPEAS

Ingredients

- 1 can (15 oz) chickpeas, drained and rinsed
- 1 tablespoon olive oil
- 1 teaspoon paprika
- 1 teaspoon garlic powder
- 1/2 teaspoon salt
- 1/4 teaspoon black pepper

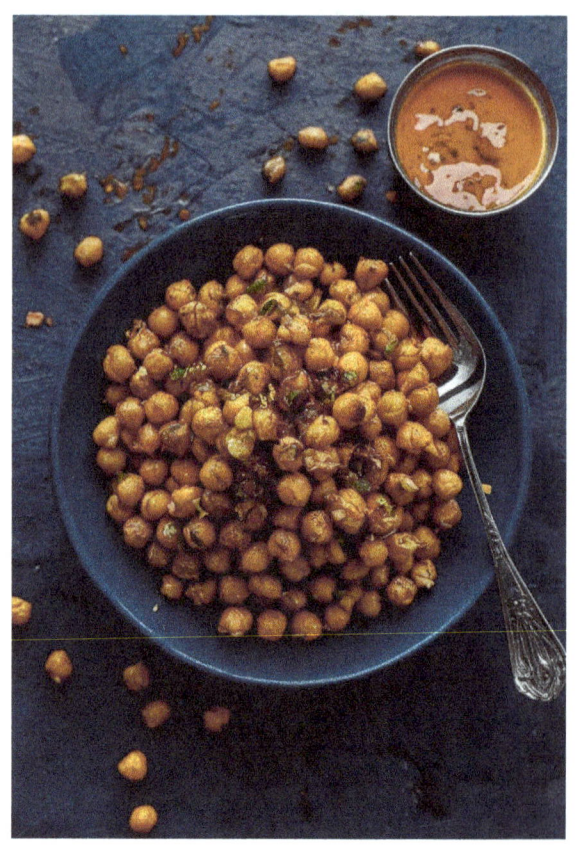

Instructions

- Preheat Oven: Preheat your oven to 400°F (200°C).
- Dry Chickpeas: Pat the chickpeas dry with paper towels.
- Season Chickpeas: In a bowl, mix chickpeas with olive oil, paprika, garlic powder, salt, and pepper.
- Bake: Spread chickpeas on a baking sheet. Bake for 35-40 minutes, shaking the pan halfway through.
- Cool: Let cool for a few minutes before serving.

 Preparation Time : 10 min

 Total Time : 50 min

 Servings : 4

Nutritional Info

- Calories: 120
- Protein: 6g
- Fat: 2g
- Carbohydrates: 20g
- Fiber: 6g

BAKED KALE CHIPS

Ingredients

- 1 bunch of kale
- 1 tablespoon olive oil (optional)
- 1 teaspoon sea salt

Instructions

- Preheat oven to 300°F (150°C).
- Prepare kale: Wash and dry kale. Tear into bite-sized pieces, removing stems.
- Season: Toss kale with olive oil (if using) and salt.
- Bake: Spread kale on a baking sheet in a single layer. Bake for 20 minutes, until edges are brown.
- Cool and serve: Let cool for a few minutes to crisp up. Enjoy!

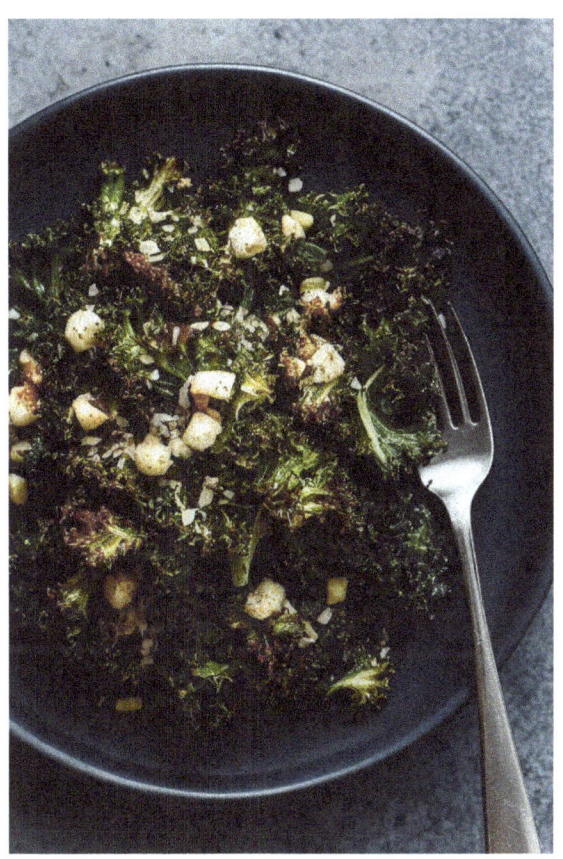

 Preparation Time : 10 min

 Total Time : 30 min

 Servings : 4

Nutritional Info

- Calories: 50
- Total Fat: 2g (with olive oil)
- Saturated Fat: 0g
- Cholesterol: 0mg
- Sodium: 200mg
- Total Carbohydrates: 8g

SPICED NUTS

Ingredients

- 2 cups mixed nuts (such as almonds, walnuts, and cashews)
- 1 tablespoon olive oil
- 1 tablespoon honey or maple syrup
- 1 teaspoon ground cinnamon
- 1/2 teaspoon ground nutmeg
- 1/4 teaspoon ground cloves
- 1/4 teaspoon salt

Instructions

- Preheat your oven to 350°F (175°C) and line a baking sheet with parchment paper.
- In a large bowl, combine the mixed nuts, olive oil, honey or maple syrup, cinnamon, nutmeg, cloves, and salt. Toss until the nuts are evenly coated.
- Spread the coated nuts in a single layer on the prepared baking sheet.
- Bake for 10-15 minutes, stirring occasionally, until the nuts are toasted and fragrant.
- Remove from the oven and let cool completely before serving or storing in an airtight container.

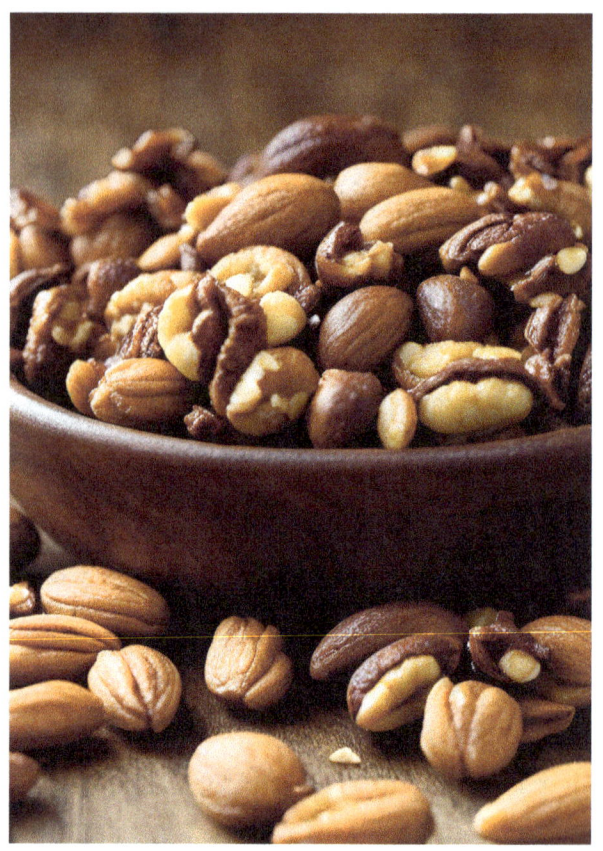

 Preparation Time : 5 min

 Total Time : 20 min

 Servings : 1/4 cup

Nutritional Info

- Calories: 180
- Protein: 5g
- Fat: 15g
- Carbohydrates: 8g
- Fiber: 2g

CRUNCHY CELERY AND APPLE SALAD

Ingredients

- 4 stalks of celery, thinly sliced
- 2 large apples (Granny Smith or Honeycrisp), cored and diced
- 1/4 cup walnuts, chopped (optional)
- 1/4 cup raisins (optional)
- 2 tablespoons lemon juice
- 1/2 teaspoon salt
- 1/4 teaspoon black pepper
- 1 tablespoon olive oil (optional)

Instructions

- Wash and thinly slice the celery stalks.
- Core and dice the apples into bite-sized pieces.
- In a large mixing bowl, combine the sliced celery and diced apples.
- If using, add the chopped walnuts and raisins to the bowl.
- Drizzle the lemon juice over the salad mixture to prevent the apples from browning.
- Season with salt and black pepper.
- Add the olive oil, if desired, for a richer flavor.
- Toss all ingredients together until well combined.
- Garnish with chopped parsley if desired.
- Serve the salad immediately to maintain its crunchiness.

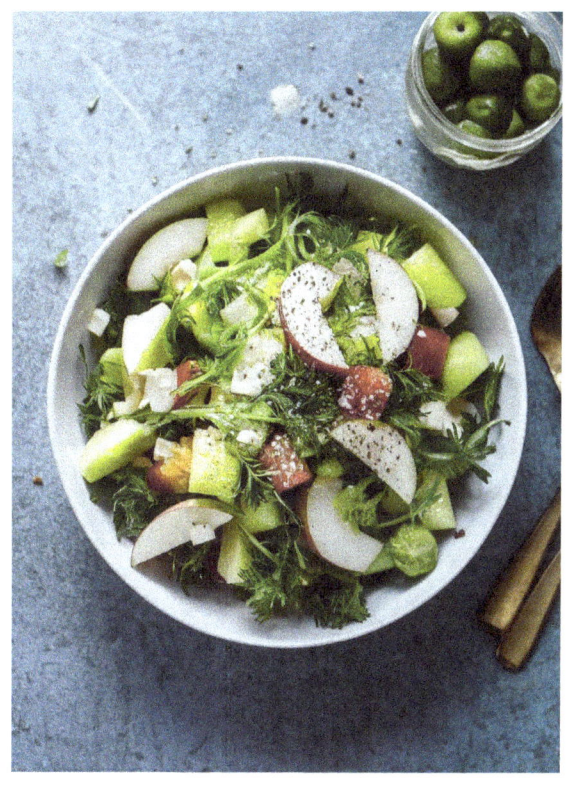

 Preparation Time : 15 min

 Total Time : 15 min

 Servings : 4

Nutritional Info

- Calories: 80
- Protein: 1g
- Carbohydrates: 18g
- Fat: 1g
- Fiber: 4g

MIXED BERRY SALAD

Ingredients

- 2 cups mixed berries (such as strawberries, blueberries, raspberries)
- 2 tablespoons honey
- 1 tablespoon balsamic vinegar
- 1/4 cup fresh mint leaves, chopped
- 1/4 cup crumbled feta cheese (optional)
- Salt and pepper to taste

Instructions

- Wash the berries and pat them dry. Slice the strawberries if they are large.
- In a small bowl, whisk together the honey and balsamic vinegar.
- In a large bowl, combine the mixed berries and chopped mint leaves.
- Drizzle the honey-balsamic dressing over the berries and gently toss to coat.
- Season with salt and pepper to taste.
- Sprinkle the crumbled feta cheese on top, if using.
- Serve immediately.

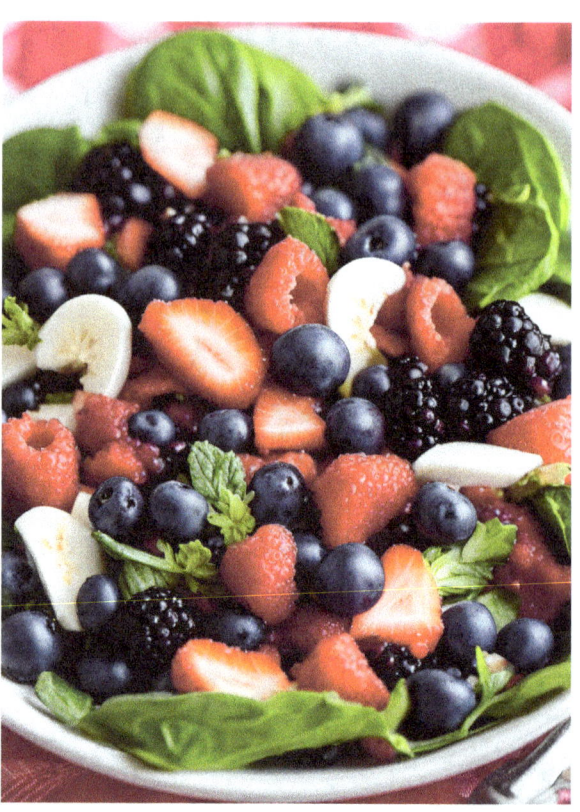

 Preparation Time : 10 min

 Total Time : 10 min

 Servings : 4

Nutritional Info

- Calories: 90
- Total Fat: 1g
- Cholesterol: 0mg
- Sodium: 20mg
- Total Carbohydrates: 22g

52

ALMOND BUTTER AND APPLE SLICES

Ingredients

- 2 medium-sized apples
- 1/4 cup almond butter
- Optional: drizzle of honey or sprinkle of cinnamon

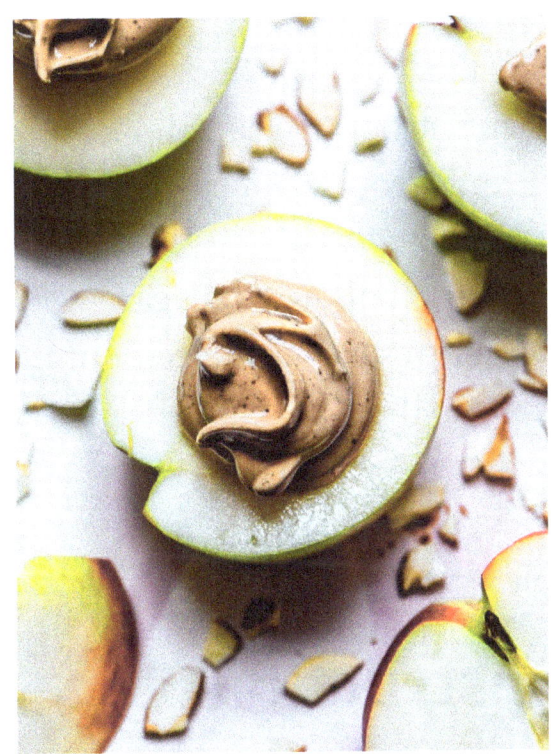

Instructions

- Wash and core the apples. Slice them into thin rounds or wedges.
- Spread almond butter on one side of each apple slice.
- Optional: Drizzle honey or sprinkle cinnamon over the almond butter.
- Serve immediately and enjoy!

Preparation Time : 5 min

Total Time : 5 min

Servings : 4

Nutritional Info

- Calories: Approximately 180 kcal
- Total Fat: 11g
- Saturated Fat: 1g
- Trans Fat: 0g
- Cholesterol: 0mg
- Sodium: 5mg

MARINATED MUSHROOM SKEWERS

Ingredients

- 1 lb (450g) button mushrooms, cleaned and stems trimmed
- 2 tbsp olive oil
- 3 tbsp balsamic vinegar
- 2 cloves garlic, minced
- 1 tsp dried thyme
- 1 tsp dried rosemary
- Salt and pepper to taste

Instructions

- Mix olive oil, balsamic vinegar, garlic, thyme, rosemary, salt, and pepper in a bowl.
- Add mushrooms and toss to coat. Let sit for 10 minutes.
- If using wooden skewers, soak them in water for 10 minutes.
- Thread mushrooms onto skewers.
- Preheat grill to medium-high.
- Grill skewers for 5-7 minutes per side, until mushrooms are tender.
- Remove from grill and enjoy warm.

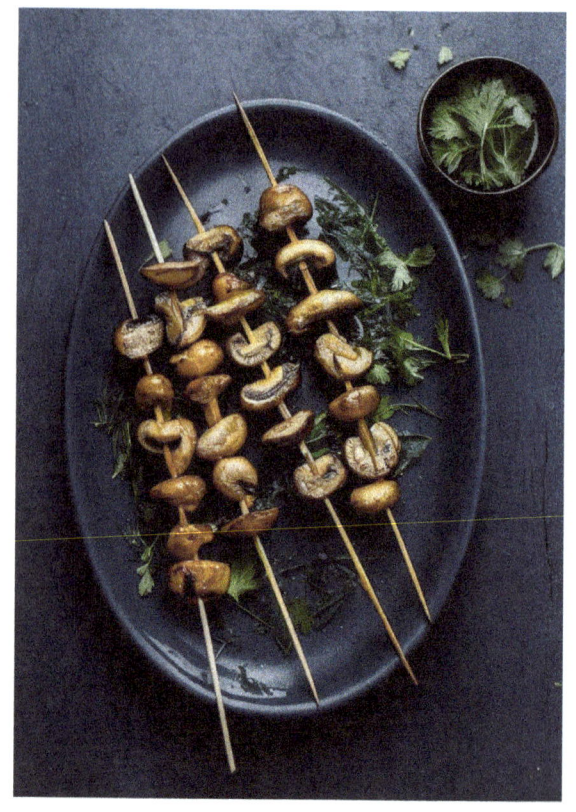

 Preparation Time : 10 min

 Total Time : 20 min

 Servings : 4

Nutritional Info

- Calories: 80
- Protein: 2g
- Carbohydrates: 6g
- Fat: 5g
- Fiber: 2g
- Sugar: 3g

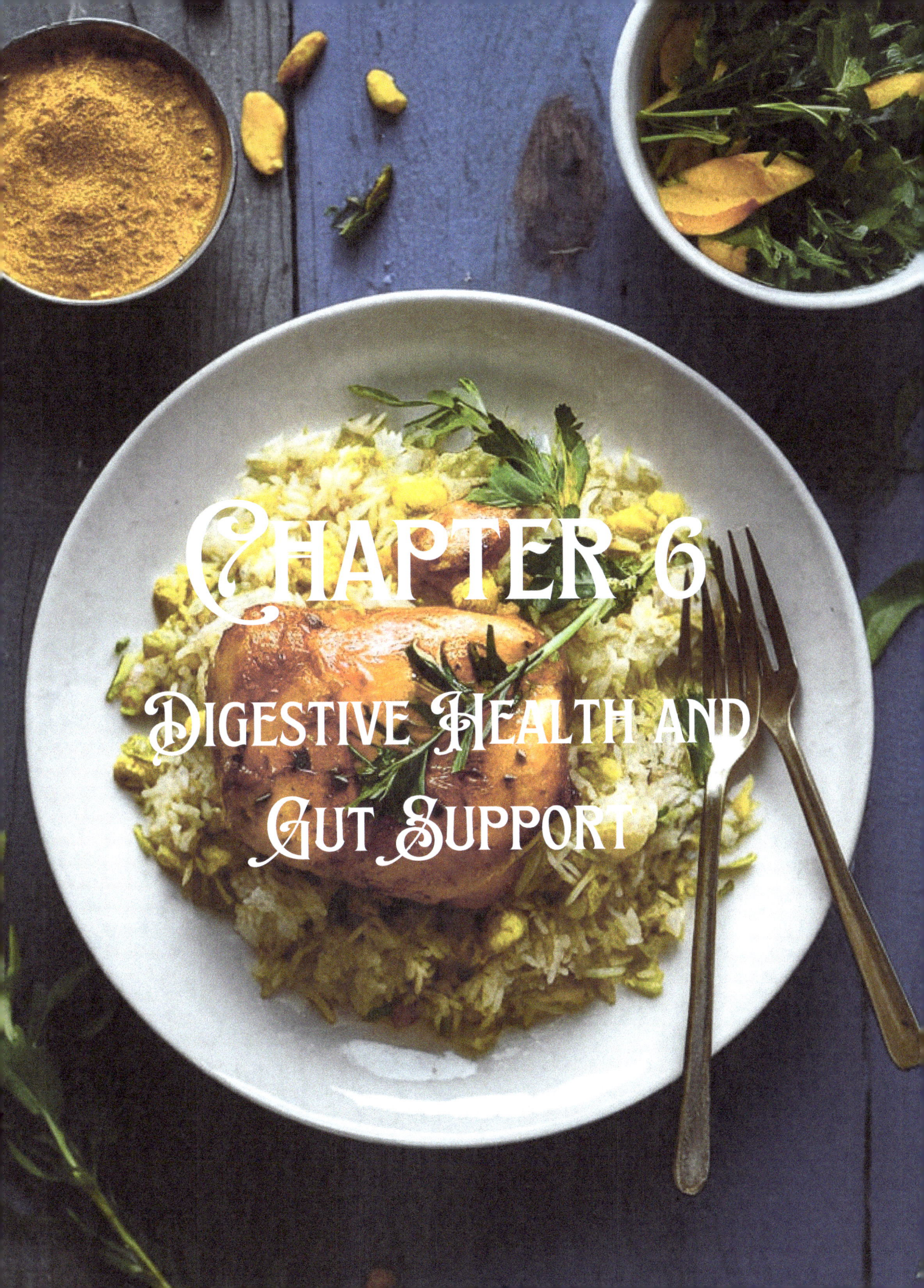

Chapter 6
Digestive Health and Gut Support

BEEF AND BROCCOLI STIR-FRY

Ingredients

- 1 lb (450g) lean beef steak, thinly sliced
- 2 cups broccoli florets
- 1 red bell pepper, thinly sliced
- 1 onion, thinly sliced
- 3 cloves garlic, minced
- 2 tbsp low-sodium soy sauce
- 1 tbsp oyster sauce
- 1 tbsp sesame oil
- 1 tbsp cornstarch
- 1 tsp fresh ginger, grated
- 2 tbsp vegetable oil
- Salt and pepper, to taste

Instructions

- In a bowl, mix soy sauce, oyster sauce, sesame oil, cornstarch, and grated ginger.
- Add beef to the marinade and let it sit for 10 minutes.
- Heat vegetable oil in a skillet or wok over medium-high heat.
- Add minced garlic and cook until fragrant, about 30 seconds.
- Add marinated beef and cook until browned, about 3 minutes. Remove beef.
- In the same skillet, add more oil if needed, then add broccoli, bell pepper, and onion. Cook for 3-4 minutes until tender-crisp.
- Return beef to the skillet, stir together, and cook for 2 minutes to heat through.
- Season with salt and pepper.
- Garnish with sesame seeds and green onions if desired.
- Serve hot over rice or noodles.

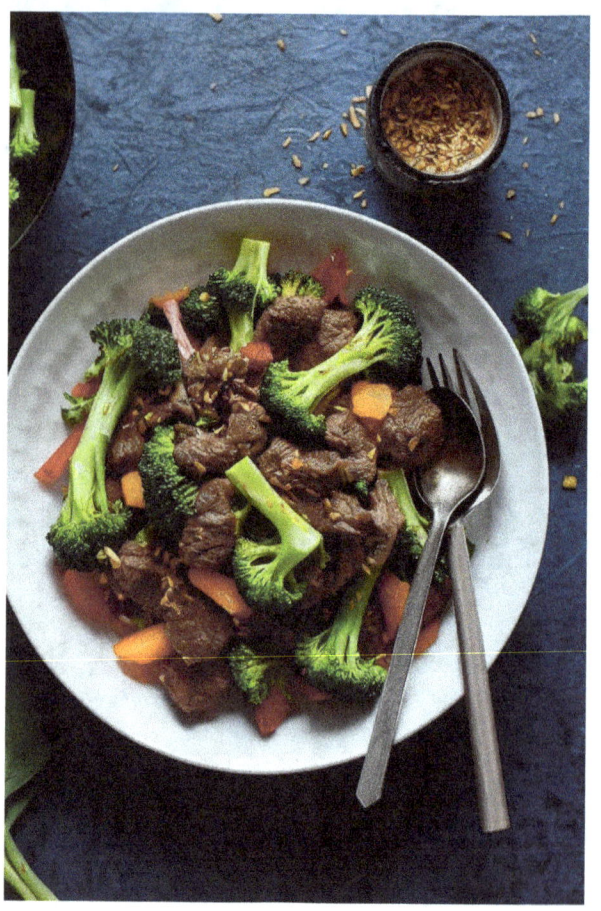

 Preparation Time : 15 min

 Total Time : 30 min

 Servings : 4

Nutritional Info

- Calories: 250
- Protein: 25g
- Carbohydrates: 12g
- Fat: 11g
- Fiber: 4g

TURKEY MEATBALLS WITH ZOODLES

Ingredients

- 1 lb ground turkey
- 1/4 cup grated Parmesan cheese
- 1 large egg
- 2 cloves garlic, minced
- 1/4 cup chopped parsley
- 1 tsp dried oregano
- 1/2 tsp salt
- 1/4 tsp black pepper
- 4 medium zucchinis, spiralized
- 2 tbsp olive oil
- 1 clove garlic, minced
- Salt and pepper to taste

Instructions

- Mix turkey, Parmesan, egg, minced garlic, parsley, oregano, salt, and pepper in a bowl.
- Shape into 1-inch meatballs.
- Heat a large skillet over medium-high heat with a bit of olive oil.
- Cook meatballs until browned and cooked through, about 10-12 minutes.
- Remove meatballs from the skillet.
- In the same skillet, heat 2 tbsp olive oil over medium heat.
- Add minced garlic and cook for 1 minute.
- Add spiralized zucchini and cook for 3-5 minutes until tender.
- Season with salt and pepper.
- Return meatballs to the skillet and add marinara sauce.
- Heat until warm.
- Serve meatballs and sauce over zoodles.

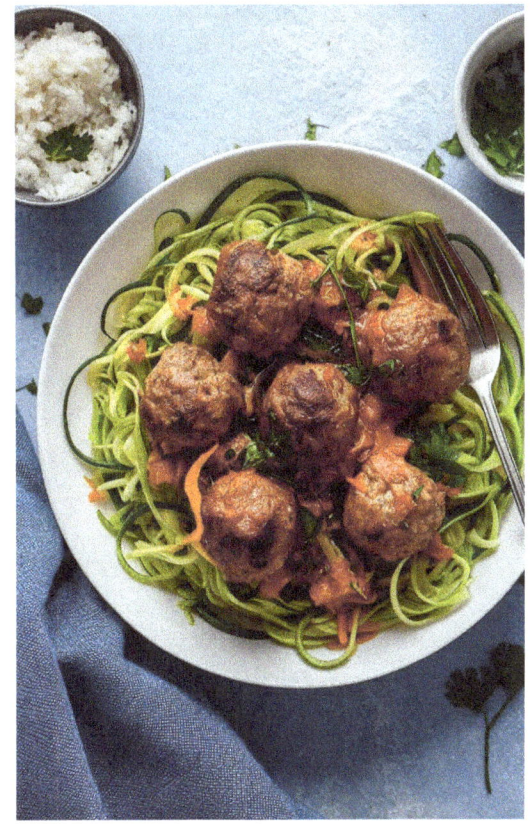

Preparation Time : 20 min

Total Time : 45 min

Servings : 4

Nutritional Info

- Calories: 250
- Protein: 30g
- Carbohydrates: 10g
- Fat: 10g
- Fiber: 3g

VEGGIE STIR-FRY WITH TOFU

Ingredients

- 1 block (14 oz) firm tofu, cubed
- 2 tablespoons soy sauce (low sodium)
- 1 tablespoon olive oil
- 2 bell peppers, sliced
- 1 cup broccoli florets
- 1 cup snap peas
- 2 cloves garlic, minced
- 1 tablespoon fresh ginger, grated
- 2 tablespoons vegetable broth (low sodium)
- Salt and pepper to taste

Instructions

- Drain, pat dry, and cube the tofu. Toss with 1 tablespoon soy sauce.
- Heat olive oil in a large pan over medium-high heat. Cook tofu until golden brown, about 5-7 minutes. Remove from pan.
- In the same pan, add garlic and ginger, sauté for 30 seconds.
- Add bell peppers, broccoli, and snap peas. Stir-fry for 4-5 minutes until tender-crisp.
- Return tofu to pan. Add 1 tablespoon soy sauce and vegetable broth. Stir and cook for 2-3 minutes.
- Season with salt and pepper. Serve warm.

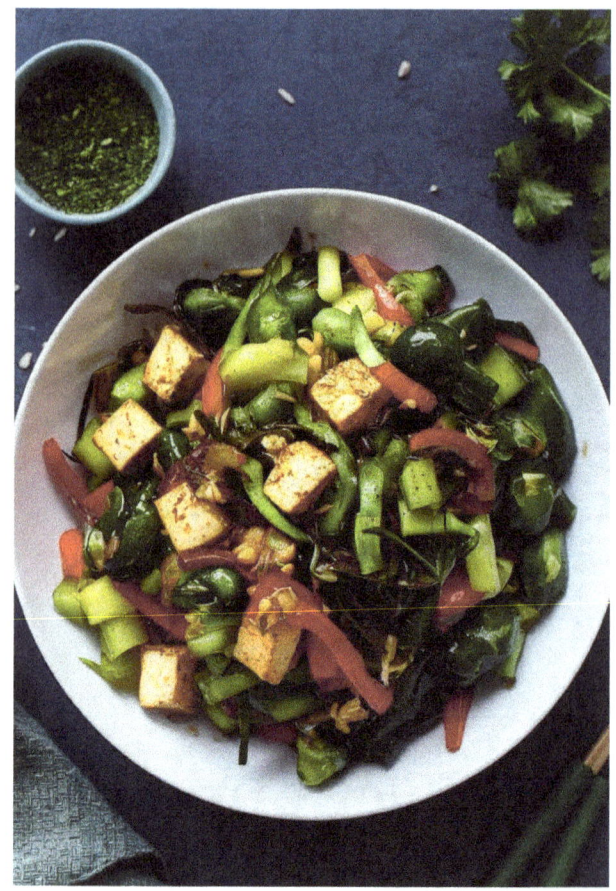

 Preparation Time : 10 min

 Total Time : 20 min

 Servings : 4

Nutritional Info

- Calories: 180
- Protein: 12g
- Carbohydrates: 16g
- Fat: 8g
- Fiber: 5g

HERB-CRUSTED CHICKEN BREAST

Ingredients

- 4 boneless, skinless chicken breasts
- 2 tablespoons olive oil
- 1/4 cup fresh parsley, chopped
- 1/4 cup fresh basil, chopped
- 1/4 cup fresh thyme, chopped
- 2 cloves garlic, minced
- 1 teaspoon salt
- 1/2 teaspoon black pepper
- 1 teaspoon lemon zest

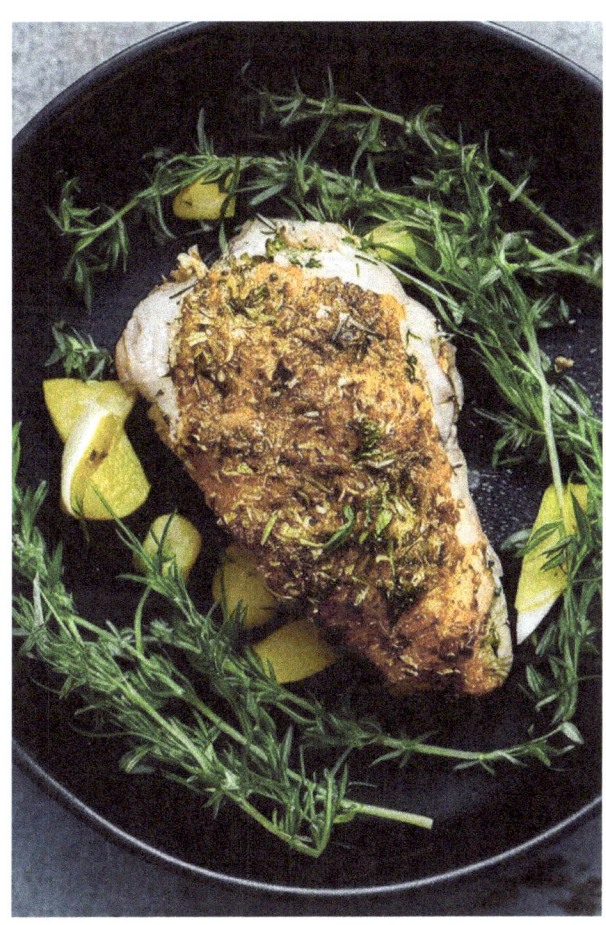

Instructions

- Preheat Oven: Preheat your oven to 400°F (200°C).
- Prepare Herb Mixture: In a small bowl, combine the chopped parsley, basil, thyme, minced garlic, salt, black pepper, and lemon zest.
- Prepare Chicken: Pat the chicken breasts dry with paper towels. Rub each breast with olive oil, ensuring they are evenly coated.
- Coat with Herbs: Press the herb mixture onto both sides of each chicken breast, making sure they are well coated.
- Bake Chicken: Place the chicken breasts on a baking sheet lined with parchment paper or in a lightly greased baking dish.
- Cook: Bake in the preheated oven for 25 minutes, or until the internal temperature of the chicken reaches 165°F (74°C) and the exterior is golden brown.
- Rest and Serve: Let the chicken rest for 5 minutes before serving to allow the juices to redistribute.

 Preparation Time : 15 min

 Total Time : 40 min

 Servings : 4

Nutritional Info

- Calories: 220
- Protein: 28g
- Carbohydrates: 2g
- Fat: 11g

SPAGHETTI SQUASH WITH MARINARA SAUCE

Ingredients

- 1 medium spaghetti squash
- 2 cups marinara sauce
- 2 tablespoons olive oil
- Salt and pepper to taste

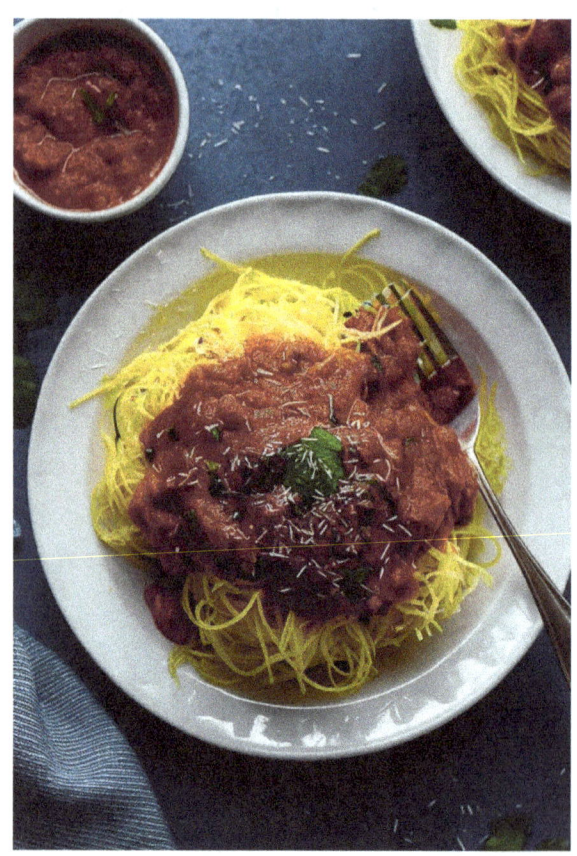

Instructions

- Preheat oven to 400°F (200°C).
- Cut spaghetti squash in half lengthwise and remove seeds.
- Drizzle olive oil over cut sides of squash and season with salt and pepper.
- Place squash halves cut-side down on a baking sheet.
- Roast squash in oven for 35-40 minutes, until tender.
- While squash is roasting, heat marinara sauce in a saucepan on medium heat.
- Once squash is done, remove from oven and let cool slightly.
- Use a fork to scrape flesh into spaghetti-like strands onto a plate.
- Pour heated marinara sauce over spaghetti squash.
- Serve hot and enjoy!

Preparation Time : 10 min

Total Time : 50 min

Servings : 4

Nutritional Info

- Calories: 150
- Total Fat: 6g
- Total Carbohydrates: 24g
- Protein: 3g

BALSAMIC GLAZED CHICKEN BREAST

Ingredients

- 4 boneless, skinless chicken breasts
- 1/2 cup balsamic vinegar
- 2 tablespoons honey
- 2 cloves garlic, minced
- 1 teaspoon dried thyme
- Salt and pepper
- 1 tablespoon olive oil

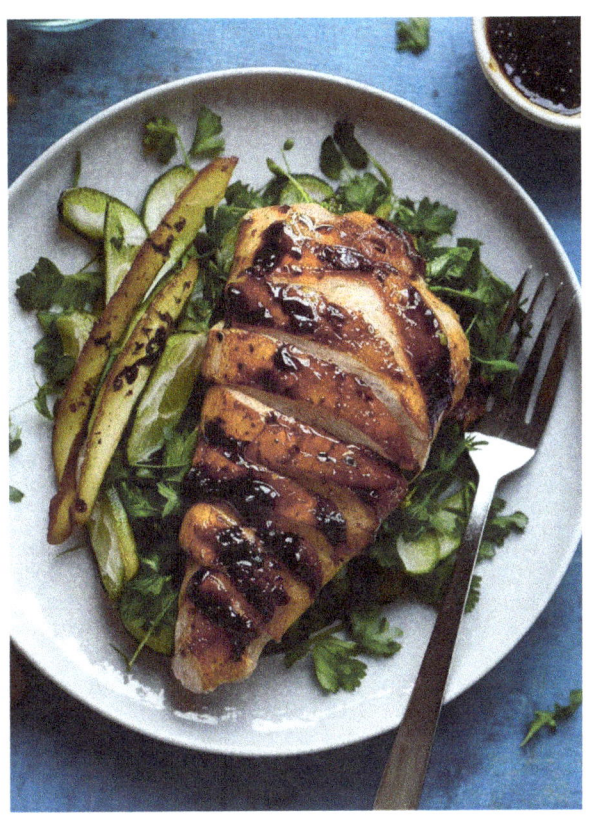

Instructions

- Mix balsamic vinegar, honey, minced garlic, and dried thyme in a bowl.
- Pour over chicken breasts and let sit for 10 minutes.
- Heat olive oil in a skillet over medium-high heat.
- Remove chicken from marinade (save marinade) and season with salt and pepper.
- Cook chicken for 5 minutes on each side until browned.
- Pour the reserved marinade into the skillet.
- Cook for another 10 minutes, turning chicken to coat with glaze, until chicken is cooked through (165°F internal temperature).
- Let chicken rest for 5 minutes.
- Drizzle with remaining glaze from the skillet.

 Preparation Time : 10 min

 Total Time : 30 min

 Servings : 4

Nutritional Info

- Calories: 200
- Protein: 30g
- Fat: 4g
- Carbohydrates: 8g

GRILLED VEGETABLE KEBABS

Ingredients

- 1 red bell pepper, cut into chunks
- 1 yellow bell pepper, cut into chunks
- 1 zucchini, sliced into rounds
- 1 red onion, cut into chunks
- 8 cherry tomatoes
- 8 button mushrooms
- 2 tablespoons olive oil
- 1 teaspoon dried oregano
- 1 teaspoon dried basil
- Salt and pepper to taste

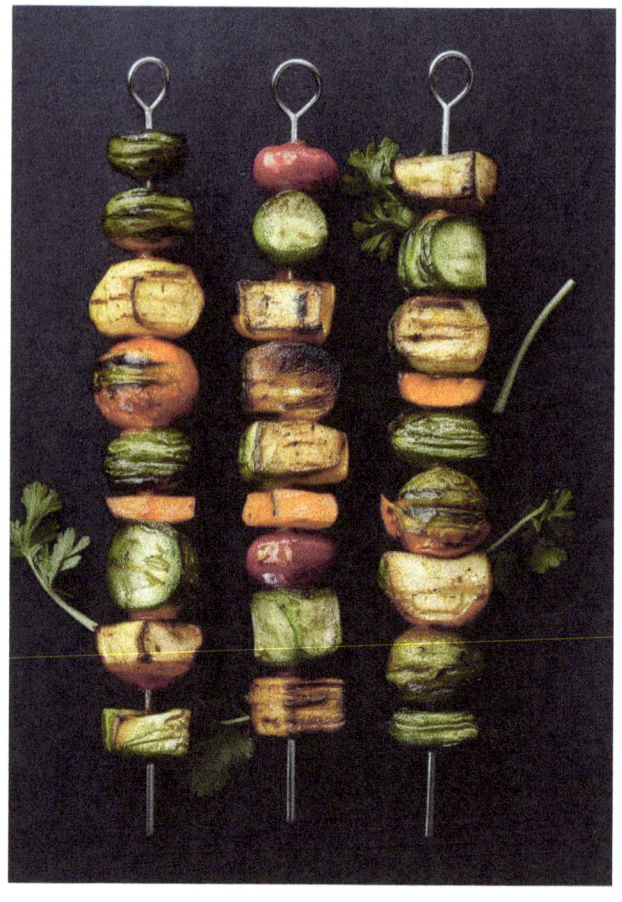

Instructions

- Wash and cut the vegetables as indicated.
- If using wooden skewers, soak them in water for at least 10 minutes to prevent burning.
- In a large bowl, combine the olive oil, dried oregano, dried basil, salt, and pepper.
- Add the cut vegetables to the bowl and toss to coat them evenly with the marinade.
- Thread the marinated vegetables onto the skewers, alternating between different types of vegetables for a colorful presentation.
- Preheat your grill to medium-high heat.
- Place the kebabs on the preheated grill.
- Grill for about 10-15 minutes, turning occasionally, until the vegetables are tender and slightly charred.
- Remove the kebabs from the grill and serve immediately.

 Preparation Time : 20 min

 Total Time : 35min

 Servings : 4

Nutritional Info

- Calories: 90
- Protein: 3g
- Carbohydrates: 15g
- Fat: 3g
- Fiber: 5g

BAKED COD WITH LEMON AND DILL

Ingredients

- 4 cod fillets (about 6 ounces each)
- 2 tablespoons olive oil
- 2 cloves garlic, minced
- 1 tablespoon fresh dill, chopped
- 1 lemon, thinly sliced
- Salt and pepper to taste

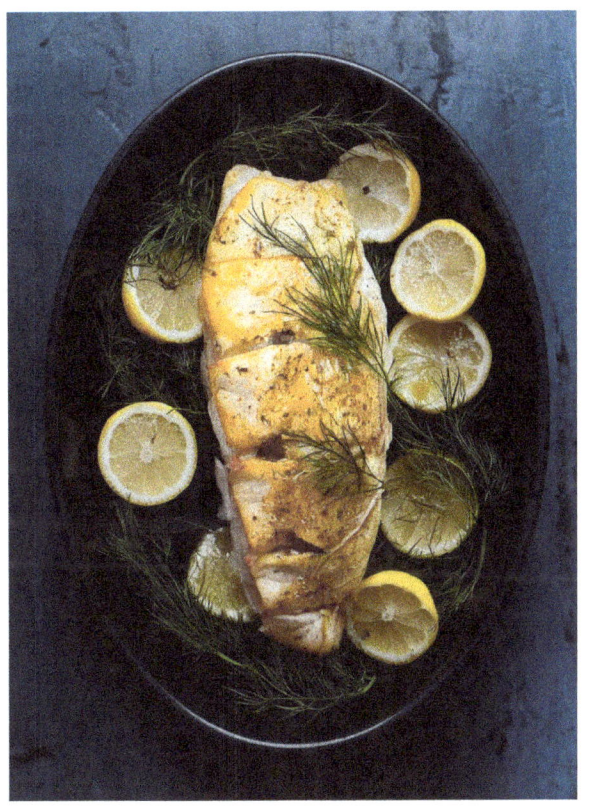

Instructions

- Preheat your oven to 375°F (190°C).
- Place the cod fillets on a baking dish lined with parchment paper or lightly greased.
- In a small bowl, mix together the olive oil, minced garlic, and chopped dill.
- Drizzle the olive oil mixture over the cod fillets, making sure they are evenly coated.
- Season the cod fillets with salt and pepper to taste.
- Place lemon slices on top of each cod fillet.
- Bake in the preheated oven for about 15-20 minutes, or until the cod is cooked through and flakes easily with a fork.
- Remove from the oven and serve hot, garnished with additional fresh dill if desired.

Preparation Time : 10 min

Total Time : 30 min

Servings : 4

Nutritional Info

- Calories: 150 kcal
- Protein: 25g
- Carbohydrates: 2g
- Fat: 4g
- Fiber: 0.5g
- Sugar: 0g

BAKED LEMON HERB SALMON

Ingredients

- 4 salmon fillets (about 6 oz each)
- 2 tablespoons olive oil
- 2 lemons (one for juice, one for slices)
- 3 cloves garlic, minced
- 2 tablespoons fresh parsley, chopped
- 1 tablespoon fresh dill, chopped
- 1 teaspoon salt
- 1/2 teaspoon black pepper

Instructions

- Preheat your oven to 400°F (200°C).
- Place the salmon fillets on a baking sheet lined with parchment paper.
- In a small bowl, mix the olive oil, juice of one lemon, minced garlic, chopped parsley, chopped dill, salt, and black pepper.
- Brush the marinade generously over each salmon fillet. Let it sit for about 10 minutes to allow the flavors to infuse.
- Slice the second lemon into thin rounds and place a couple of slices on top of each salmon fillet.
- Bake in the preheated oven for 20 minutes, or until the salmon is cooked through and flakes easily with a fork.
- Remove from the oven and transfer to plates. Serve immediately, optionally garnished with extra fresh herbs and lemon wedges.

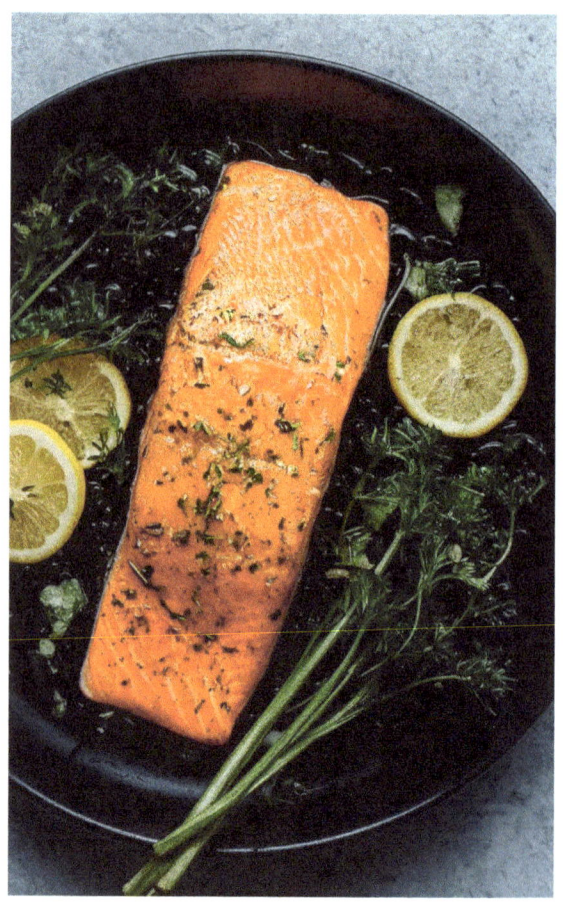

 Preparation Time : 10 min

 Total Time : 30 min

 Servings : 4

Nutritional Info

- Calories: 230
- Protein: 25g
- Fat: 14g
- Carbohydrates: 2g
- Fiber: 1g

GRILLED SHRIMP SKEWERS

Ingredients

- 1 lb large shrimp, peeled and deveined
- 2 cloves garlic, minced
- 2 tbsp olive oil
- 1 tbsp lemon juice
- 1 tsp smoked paprika
- Salt and pepper to taste
- Fresh parsley, chopped (for garnish)

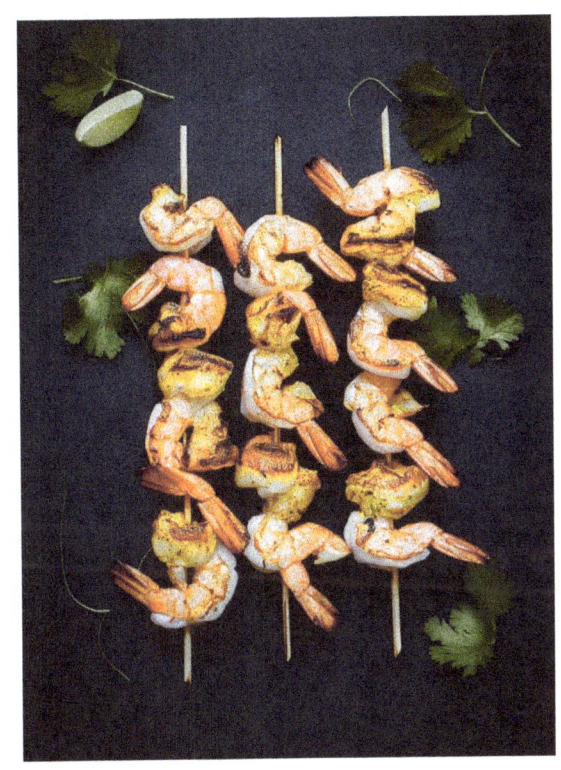

Instructions

- Marinate the Shrimp: In a large bowl, combine minced garlic, olive oil, lemon juice, smoked paprika, salt, and pepper. Add the shrimp and toss to coat. Let it marinate for 10 minutes.
- Prepare the Skewers: If using wooden skewers, soak them in water for 10 minutes to prevent burning. Thread the shrimp onto the skewers, leaving a little space between each shrimp.
- Preheat the Grill: Preheat the grill to medium-high heat.
- Grill the Shrimp: Place the shrimp skewers on the grill. Cook for 2-3 minutes per side, until the shrimp are opaque and cooked through.
- Serve: Remove the skewers from the grill and transfer to a serving platter. Garnish with chopped fresh parsley and lemon wedges. Serve immediately.

 Preparation Time : 15 min

 Total Time : 25 min

 Servings : 4

Nutritional Info

- Calories: 150
- Protein: 23g
- Carbohydrates: 2g
- Fat: 6g
- Fiber: 0g

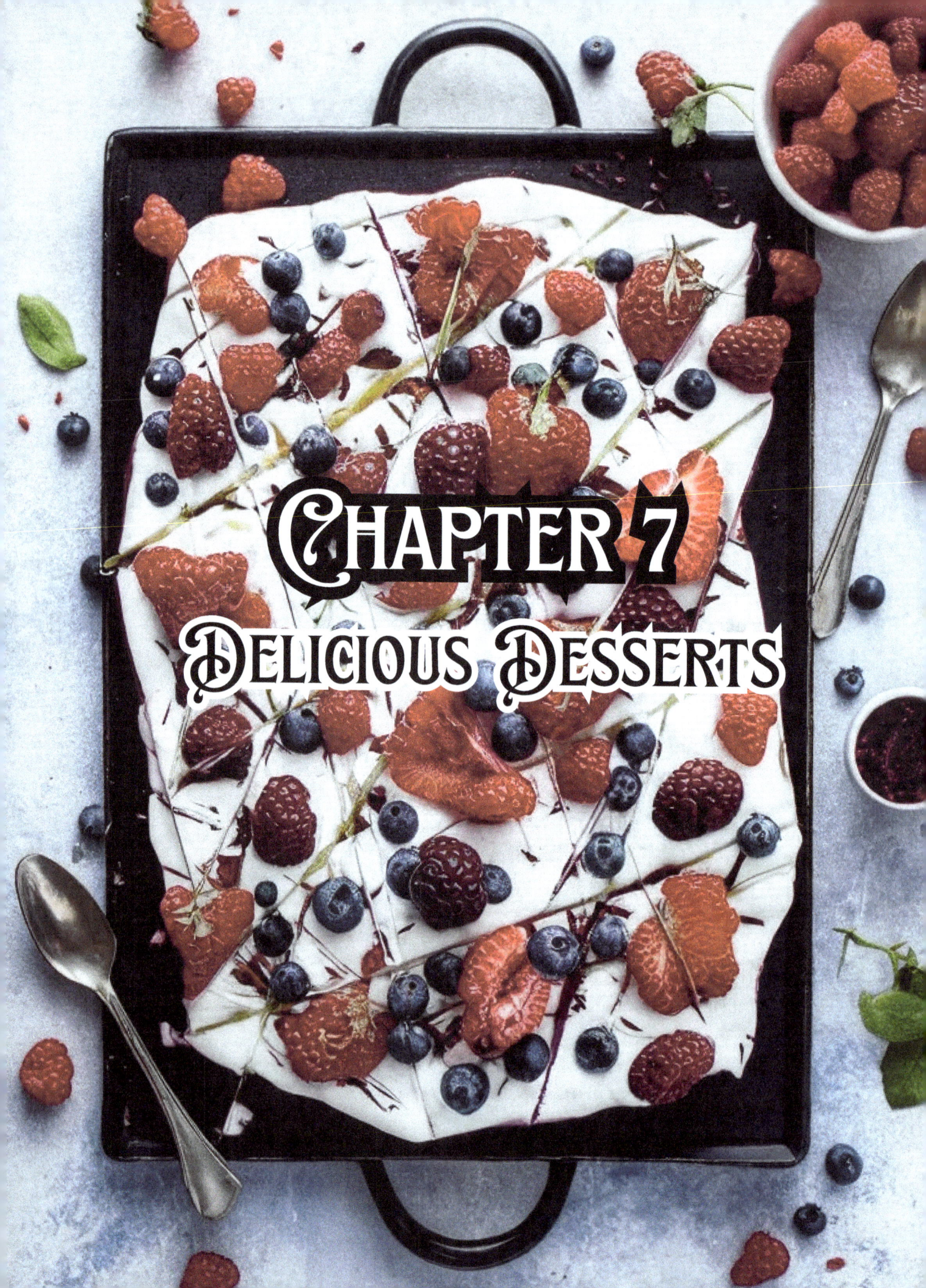

Chapter 7
Delicious Desserts

MIXED BERRY SORBET

Ingredients

- 3 cups mixed berries (such as strawberries, blueberries, raspberries)
- 1/4 cup honey or maple syrup (optional)
- 2 tablespoons lemon juice

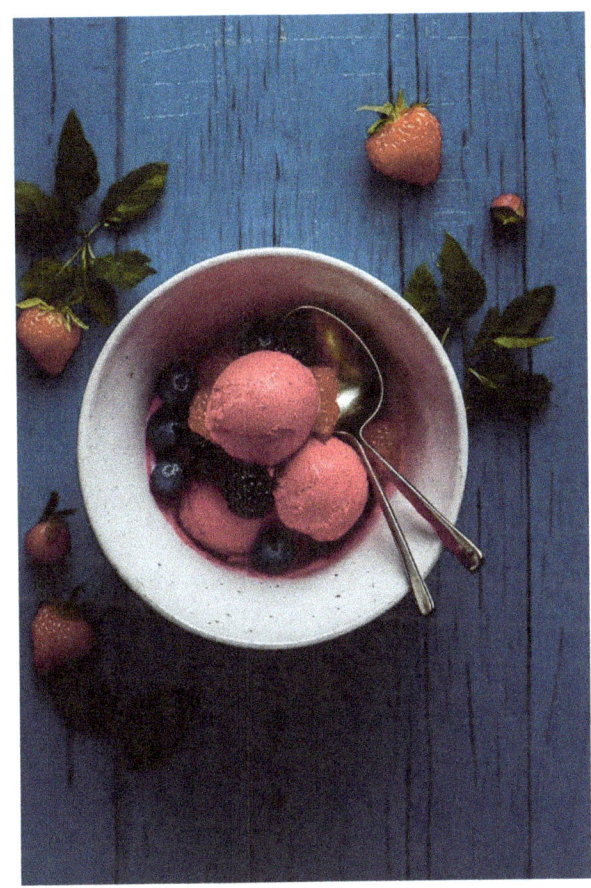

Preparation Time : 10 min

Total Time : 0 min

Servings : 4

Instructions

- Blend: Put the mixed berries, honey or maple syrup (if using), and lemon juice in a blender or food processor.
- Blend Again: Blend until smooth.
- Freeze: Pour the mixture into a shallow dish or pan. Cover and freeze for 3-4 hours, or until partially frozen.
- Scrape and Blend: Once partially frozen, scrape the mixture with a fork to break it up into icy flakes. Blend again until smooth.
- Freeze Again: Return the mixture to the dish or pan. Cover and freeze for another 2-3 hours, or until firm.
- Serve: Scoop the sorbet into bowls or glasses.
- Enjoy: Garnish with fresh mint leaves if desired, then serve and enjoy!

Nutritional Info

- Calories: Approximately 80 kcal
- Carbohydrates: Approximately 20 g
- Fiber: Approximately 3 g
- Sugars: Approximately 15 g
- Fat: Approximately 0 g

APPLE CINNAMON COMPOTE

Ingredients

- 4 medium apples, peeled, cored, and chopped
- 1 tablespoon lemon juice
- 1/4 cup water
- 2 tablespoons honey or maple syrup (optional)
- 1 teaspoon ground cinnamon
- 1/2 teaspoon vanilla extract (optional)

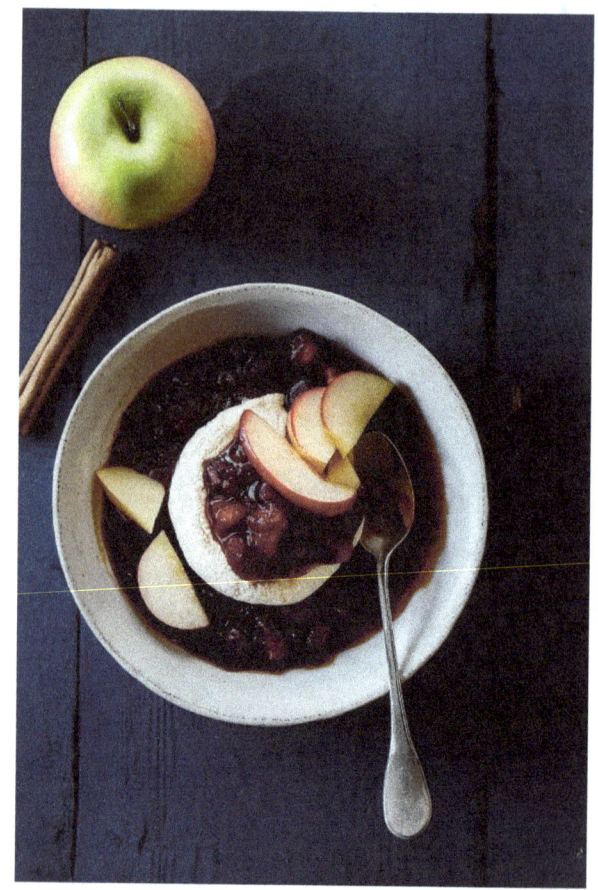

Instructions

- In a medium saucepan, combine the chopped apples, lemon juice, and water.
- Bring the mixture to a simmer over medium heat.
- Stir in the honey or maple syrup (if using), ground cinnamon, and vanilla extract (if using).
- Reduce the heat to low and let the mixture cook uncovered for about 15-20 minutes, or until the apples are soft and the liquid has thickened slightly, stirring occasionally.
- Once the apples are cooked to your desired consistency, remove the saucepan from the heat.
- Allow the compote to cool slightly before serving. You can serve it warm or chilled, depending on your preference.
- Enjoy the apple cinnamon compote on its own, or use it as a topping for yogurt, oatmeal, pancakes, or ice cream.

 Preparation Time : 10 min

 Total Time : 30 min

 Servings : 4

Nutritional Info

- Calories: 80 kcal
- Carbohydrates: 20 g
- Fiber: 4 g
- Sugars: 15 g
- Fat: 0 g
- Protein: 0 g

PEACH AND RASPBERRY CRUMBLE

Ingredients

- 1 ripe peach, sliced
- 1/2 cup fresh raspberries
- 1 tablespoon lemon juice
- 2 tablespoons granulated sugar (or sweetener of choice)
- 1/4 cup rolled oats
- 2 tablespoons all-purpose flour
- 1 tablespoon brown sugar
- 1/4 teaspoon ground cinnamon
- 2 tablespoons unsalted butter, chilled and cubed

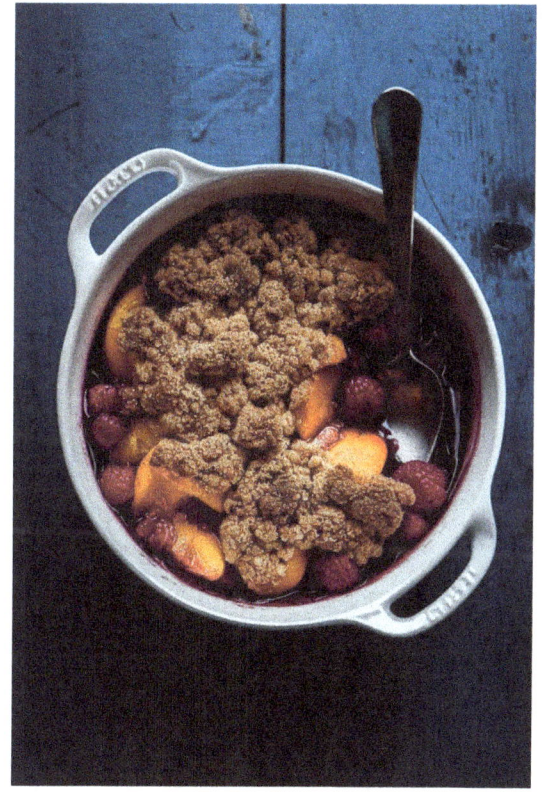

Instructions

- Preheat your oven to 375°F (190°C). Lightly grease a small baking dish or individual ramekins.
- In a bowl, toss together the sliced peach, raspberries, lemon juice, and granulated sugar until well combined. Transfer the fruit mixture to the prepared baking dish or ramekins, spreading it out evenly.
- In another bowl, mix together the rolled oats, all-purpose flour, brown sugar, and ground cinnamon.
- Using your fingers, incorporate the chilled cubed butter into the oat mixture until it resembles coarse crumbs.
- Sprinkle the oat mixture evenly over the fruit in the baking dish or ramekins.
- Place the baking dish or ramekins in the preheated oven and bake for about 25-30 minutes, or until the fruit is bubbly and the crumble topping is golden brown.
- Remove from the oven and let it cool for a few minutes before serving.
- Serve warm as is or with a scoop of vanilla frozen yogurt or a dollop of whipped cream, if desired.

 Preparation Time : 15 min

 Total Time : 45 min

 Servings : 1

Nutritional Info

- Calories: 250 kcal
- Carbohydrates: 40g
- Protein: 3g
- Fat: 10g
- Fiber: 5g

BAKED APPLES WITH CINNAMON

Ingredients

- 4 medium-sized apples
- 1 teaspoon ground cinnamon

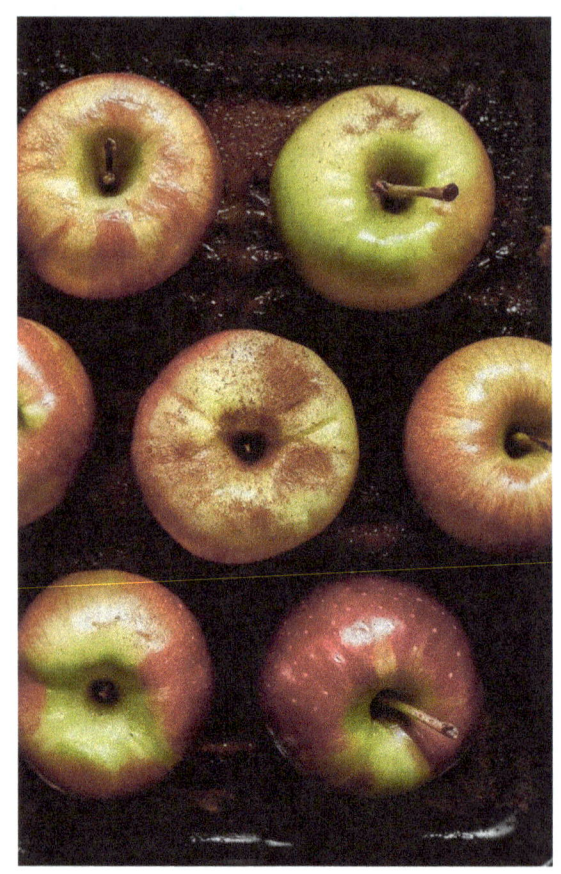

Instructions

- Preheat your oven to 375°F (190°C).
- Wash the apples and remove the cores, leaving the bottoms intact to hold the filling.
- Place the cored apples in a baking dish.
- Sprinkle ground cinnamon evenly over each apple.
- Bake for 25 minutes, or until the apples are tender.
- Serve warm as is or with a dollop of Greek yogurt or a scoop of vanilla ice cream, if desired.

Preparation Time : 5 min

Total Time : 30 min

Servings : 4

Nutritional Info

- Calories: 120 kcal
- Total Fat: 0.5g
- Carbohydrates: 31g
- Fiber: 5g
- Sugars: 24g
- Protein: 0.5g

BLUEBERRY AND LEMON SORBET

Ingredients

- 2 cups fresh blueberries
- 1/2 cup water
- 1/2 cup granulated sugar
- Zest and juice of 1 lemon

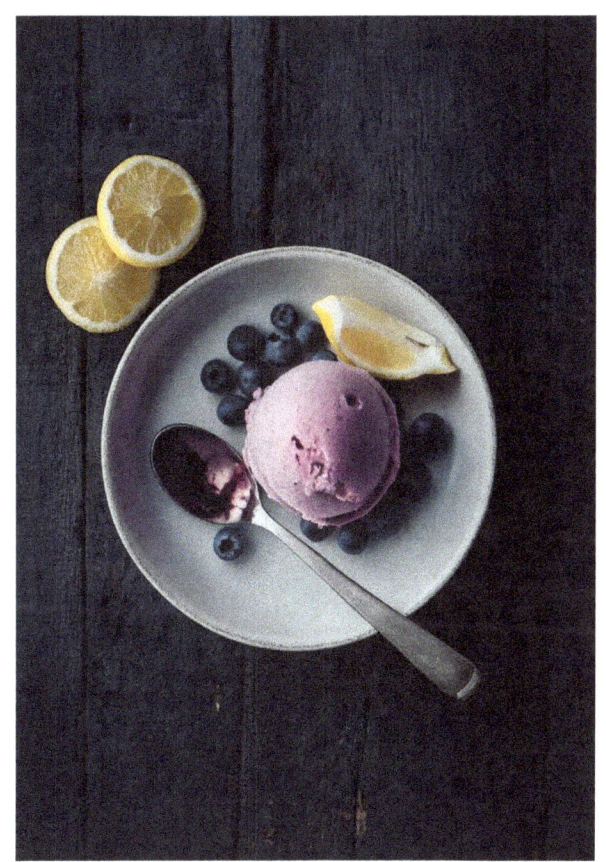

Instructions

- Combine Ingredients: In a saucepan, mix blueberries, water, and sugar. Heat on medium until sugar dissolves and blueberries soften (about 5 minutes).
- Blend: Pour mixture into a blender, add lemon zest and juice, blend until smooth.
- Strain (Optional): If desired, strain mixture through a sieve for smoother texture.
- Chill and Freeze: Cool mixture in the fridge for 2 hours. Pour into a shallow dish, freeze for 4-6 hours. Stir every hour.
- Serve: Scoop into bowls, garnish with blueberries or lemon zest. Enjoy!

Preparation Time : 10 min

Total Time : 15 min

Servings : 4

Nutritional Info

- Calories: 80 kcal
- Fat: 0g
- Carbohydrates: 20g
- Fiber: 3g
- Sugars: 14g
- Protein: 1g

MANGO AND PINEAPPLE SALAD

Ingredients

- 1 ripe mango, peeled and diced
- 1 cup fresh pineapple chunks
- 1/4 cup red onion, finely chopped
- 1/4 cup fresh cilantro, chopped
- Juice of 1 lime
- Salt and pepper to taste

Instructions

- In a large mixing bowl, combine the diced mango, pineapple chunks, chopped red onion, and chopped cilantro.
- Squeeze the lime juice over the fruit mixture.
- Season with salt and pepper to taste.
- Gently toss the ingredients until everything is evenly coated with lime juice and seasoning.
- Serve immediately as a refreshing side dish or as a topping for grilled chicken or fish.

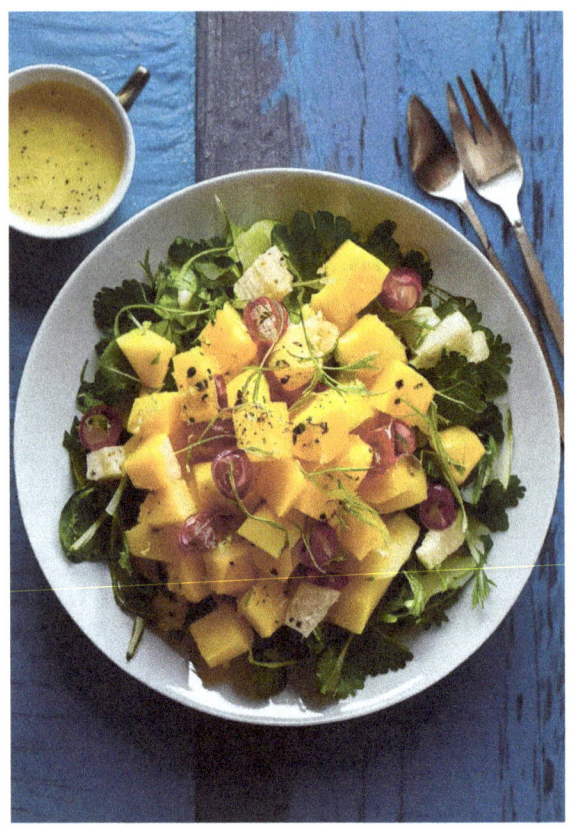

Preparation Time : 10 min

Total Time : 0 min

Servings : 4

Nutritional Info

- Calories: 80 kcal
- Protein: 1g
- Carbohydrates: 21g
- Fat: 0g
- Fiber: 3g
- Sugar: 16g
- Sodium: 5mg

FROZEN YOGURT BARK WITH BERRIES

Ingredients

- 2 cups plain Greek yogurt
- 2 tablespoons honey or maple syrup
- 1 teaspoon vanilla extract
- 1 cup mixed berries (such as strawberries, blueberries, and raspberries)
- Optional: 2 tablespoons shredded coconut or chopped nuts for toppin

Instructions

- In a mixing bowl, combine the Greek yogurt, honey (or maple syrup), and vanilla extract. Stir until well combined.
- Line a baking sheet with parchment paper or a silicone baking mat.
- Pour the yogurt mixture onto the prepared baking sheet, spreading it evenly to about ¼ inch thickness.
- Scatter the mixed berries evenly over the yogurt mixture. Press them gently into the yogurt.
- If desired, sprinkle shredded coconut or chopped nuts over the top for added texture and flavor.
- Place the baking sheet in the freezer and let the yogurt bark freeze for at least 2 hours, or until completely firm.
- Once frozen, remove the baking sheet from the freezer and break the yogurt bark into pieces using your hands or a knife.
- Serve immediately as a refreshing snack or dessert. Store any leftovers in an airtight container in the freezer.

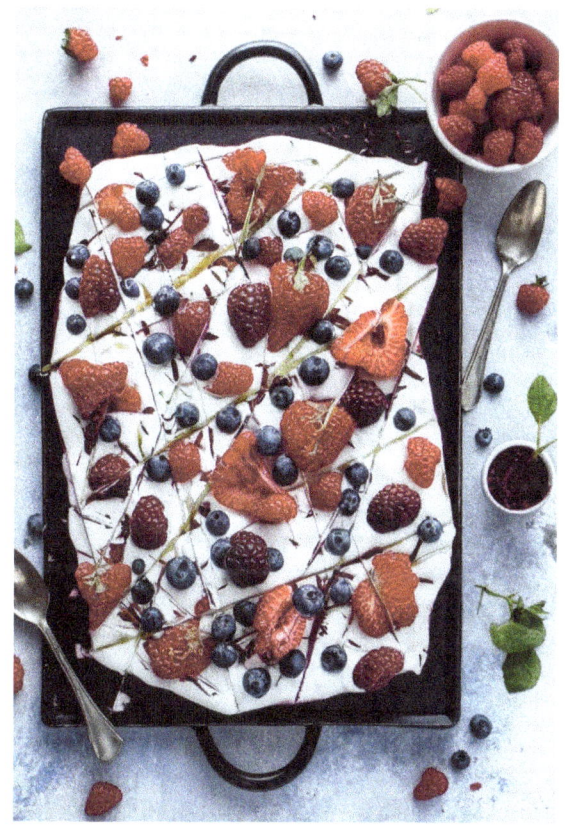

Preparation Time : 10 min

Total Time : 2hrs 10 min

Servings : 6

Nutritional Info

- Calories: 110 kcal
- Total Fat: 2g
- Saturated Fat: 1g
- Cholesterol: 5mg
- Sodium: 25mg
- Total Carbohydrates: 14g

CHOCOLATE DIPPED STRAWBERRIES

Ingredients

- 1 pint of fresh strawberries, washed and dried
- 4 oz (about 120g) of dark chocolate chips or chopped dark chocolate (70% cocoa or higher)

Instructions

- Line a baking sheet with parchment paper.
- In a microwave-safe bowl, melt the dark chocolate chips in 30-second intervals, stirring in between, until smooth and fully melted.
- Hold each strawberry by the stem and dip it into the melted chocolate, swirling to coat it partially.
- Place the dipped strawberries onto the prepared baking sheet.
- Repeat with the remaining strawberries.
- Place the baking sheet in the refrigerator for about 15-20 minutes or until the chocolate sets.
- Once the chocolate has hardened, transfer the chocolate-dipped strawberries to a serving plate.
- Serve immediately as a delicious and healthy dessert option.

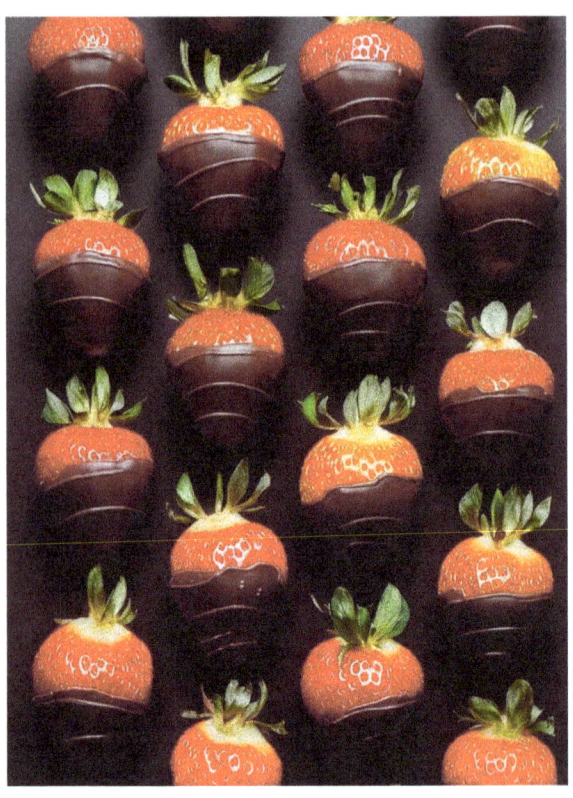

Preparation Time : 10 min

Total Time : 15 min

Servings : 4

Nutritional Info

- Calories: 120
- Total Fat: 7g
- Saturated Fat: 4g
- Cholesterol: 0mg
- Sodium: 5mg
- Total Carbohydrates: 15g

GRILLED PINEAPPLE WITH CINNAMON

Ingredients

- 1 ripe pineapple, peeled and cored
- 1 teaspoon ground cinnamon

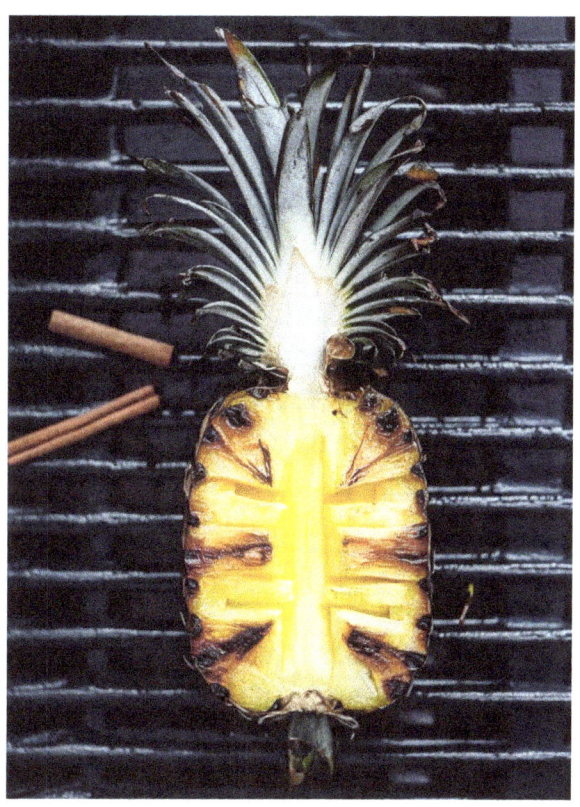

Instructions

- Preheat your grill to medium-high heat.
- Slice the pineapple into rings or wedges, about 1/2 inch thick.
- Sprinkle both sides of the pineapple slices with ground cinnamon.
- Place the pineapple slices on the preheated grill.
- Grill for 3-4 minutes on each side, or until grill marks appear and the pineapple is heated through.
- Remove from the grill and serve hot.

 Preparation Time : 10 min

 Total Time : 5 min

 Servings : 2

Nutritional Info

- Calories: 90
- Total Fat: 0g
- Saturated Fat: 0g
- Cholesterol: 0mg
- Sodium: 0mg
- Total Carbohydrates: 23g

COCONUT MACAROONS

Ingredients

- 3 cups shredded coconut
- 3/4 cup sweetened condensed milk
- 2 large egg whites
- 1 teaspoon vanilla extract
- Pinch of salt

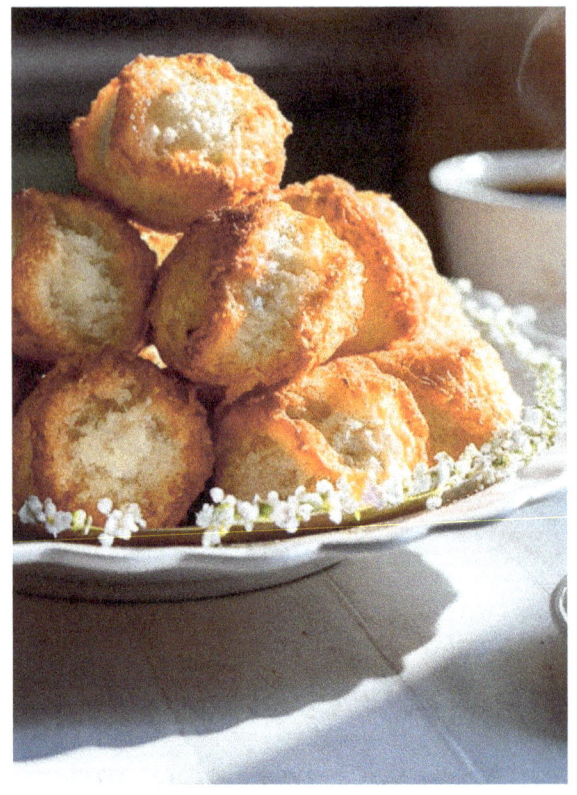

Instructions

- Preheat your oven to 325°F (160°C). Line a baking sheet with parchment paper.
- In a large bowl, combine the shredded coconut, sweetened condensed milk, vanilla extract, and salt. Mix well until evenly combined.
- In a separate bowl, beat the egg whites until stiff peaks form.
- Gently fold the beaten egg whites into the coconut mixture until fully incorporated.
- Using a spoon or cookie scoop, drop rounded tablespoons of the mixture onto the prepared baking sheet, spacing them about 1 inch apart.
- Bake in the preheated oven for 20-25 minutes, or until the macaroons are golden brown on the edges.
- Remove from the oven and let cool on the baking sheet for a few minutes before transferring to a wire rack to cool completely.

Preparation Time : 10 min

Total Time : 35 min

Servings : 20 macaroons

Nutritional Info

- Calories: 120 kcal
- Total Fat: 7g
- Saturated Fat: 6g
- Trans Fat: 0g
- Cholesterol: 3mg
- Sodium: 60mg

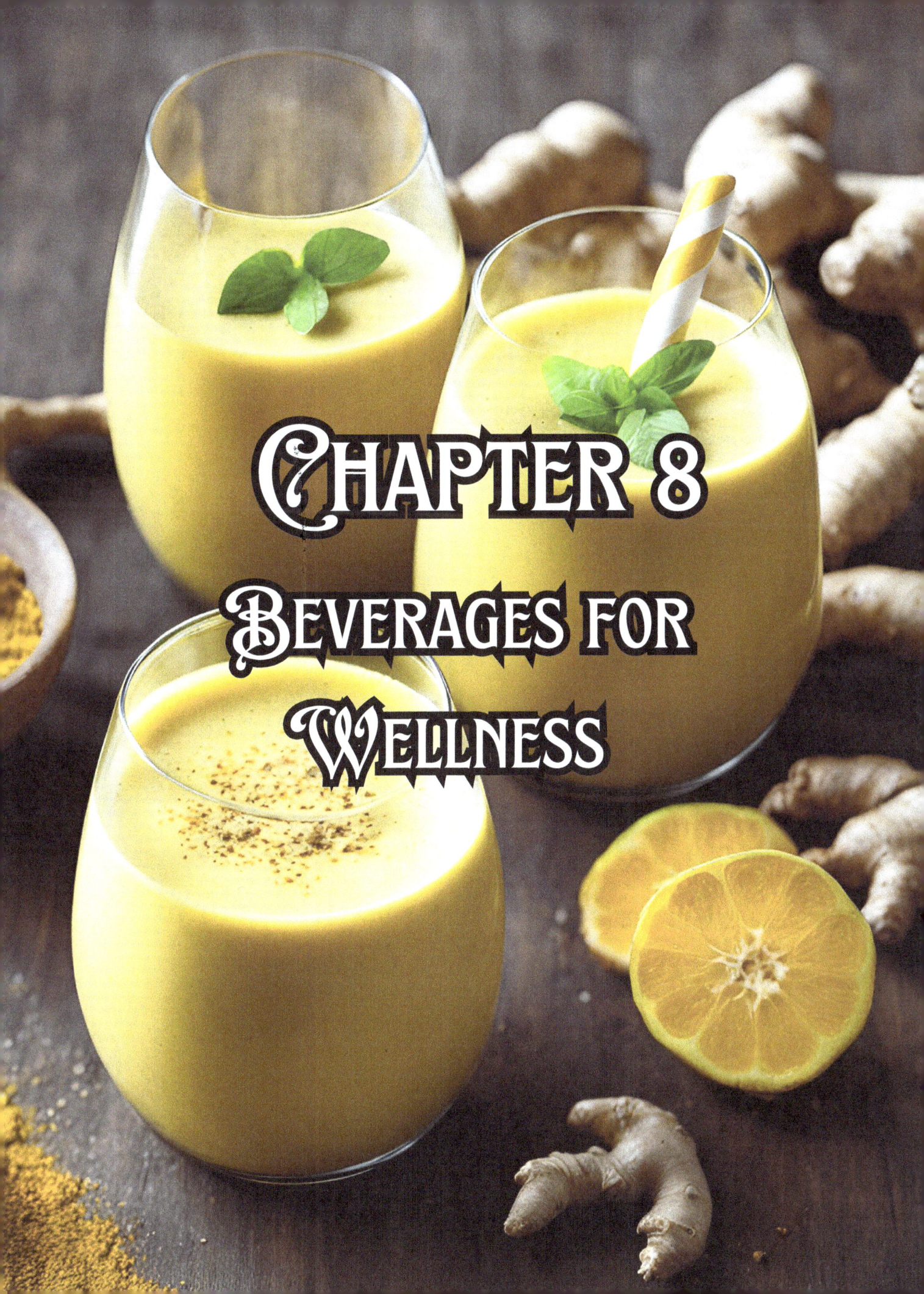

Chapter 8
Beverages for Wellness

WATERMELON COOLER

Ingredients

- 2 cups of diced seedless watermelon
- 1/2 cup of fresh lime juice
- 1 tablespoon of honey or agave syrup (optional)
- Ice cubes
- Fresh mint leaves for garnish (optional)

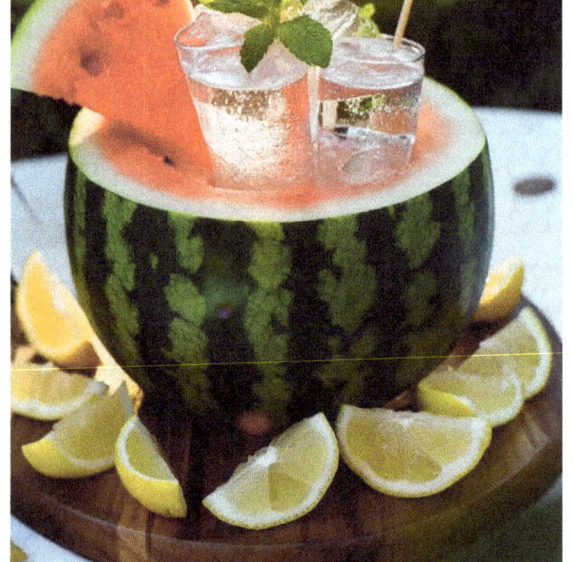

Instructions

- In a blender, combine the diced watermelon, lime juice, and honey (if using).
- Blend until smooth and well combined.
- Taste and adjust sweetness if necessary by adding more honey.
- Fill a glass with ice cubes.
- Pour the watermelon mixture over the ice cubes.
- Garnish with fresh mint leaves if desired.
- Serve immediately and enjoy!

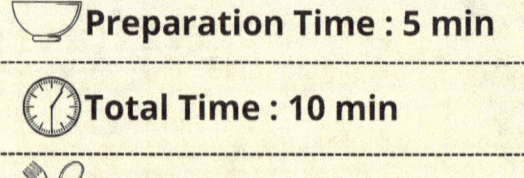

Preparation Time : 5 min

Total Time : 10 min

Servings : 1

Nutritional Info

- Calories: 70 kcal
- Total Fat: 0 g
- Saturated Fat: 0 g
- Cholesterol: 0 mg
- Sodium: 2 mg
- Total Carbohydrates: 18 g

CUCUMBER MINT WATER

Ingredients

- 1 medium cucumber, thinly sliced
- 1/4 cup fresh mint leaves
- 1 lemon, thinly sliced
- 4 cups cold water
- Ice cubes (optional)

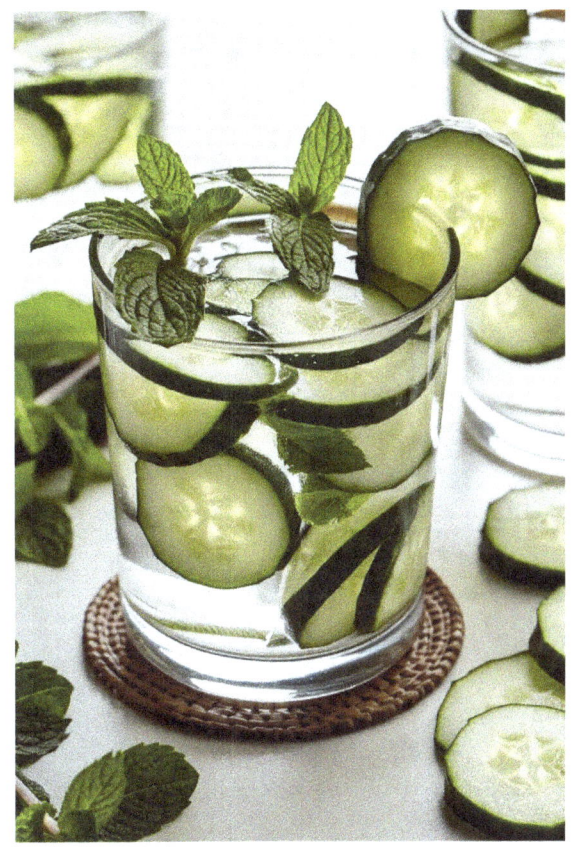

Instructions

- In a large pitcher, add the sliced cucumber, fresh mint leaves, and lemon slices.
- Pour cold water over the ingredients in the pitcher.
- Stir gently to combine.
- Refrigerate the cucumber mint water for at least 1 hour to allow the flavors to infuse.
- Serve chilled over ice cubes, if desired.

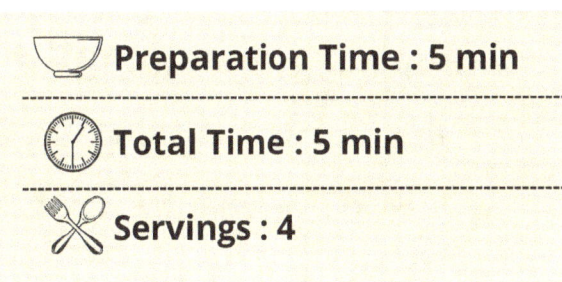

Preparation Time : 5 min

Total Time : 5 min

Servings : 4

Nutritional Info

- Calories: 4
- Total Fat: 0g
- Cholesterol: 0mg
- Sodium: 2mg
- Total Carbohydrates: 1g
- Dietary Fiber: 0g

LEMON LIME INFUSION

Ingredients

- 1 lemon, thinly sliced
- 1 lime, thinly sliced
- Ice cubes (optional)
- Water

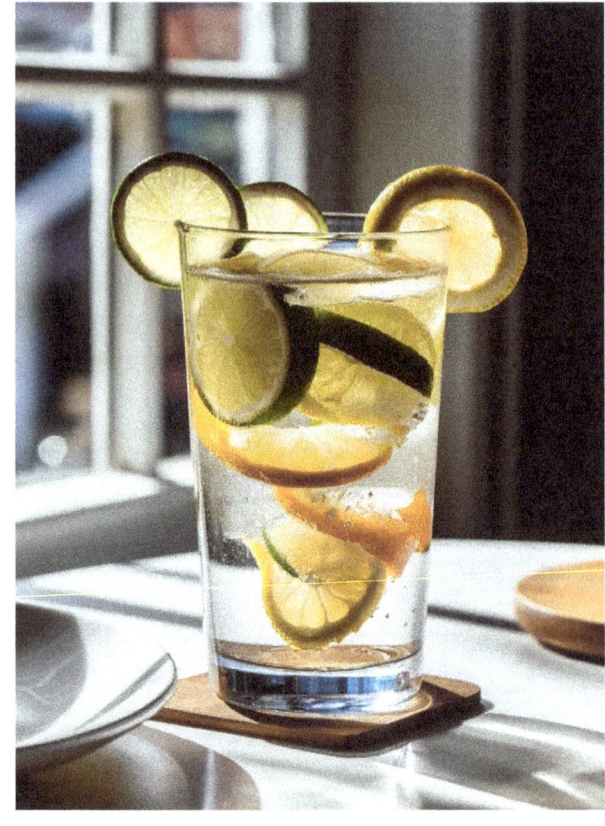

Instructions

- Place lemon and lime slices into a pitcher.
- Add ice cubes if desired.
- Fill the pitcher with water.
- Allow the water to infuse for at least 30 minutes before serving.
- Serve chilled and enjoy!

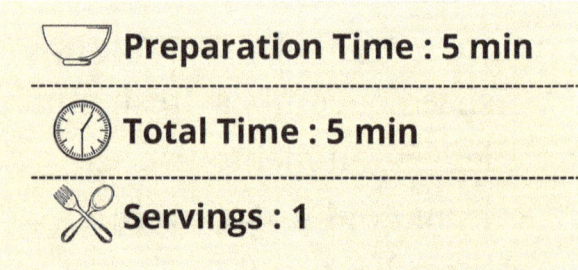

Preparation Time : 5 min

Total Time : 5 min

Servings : 1

Nutritional Info

- Calories: 0
- Carbohydrates: 0g
- Fat: 0g
- Protein: 0g

TROPICAL FRUIT SMOOTHIE

Ingredients

- 1/2 cup frozen pineapple chunks
- 1/2 cup frozen mango chunks
- 1/2 cup frozen banana slices
- 1/2 cup coconut water
- 1/4 cup Greek yogurt
- 1 tablespoon honey (optional)
- Juice of 1/2 lime

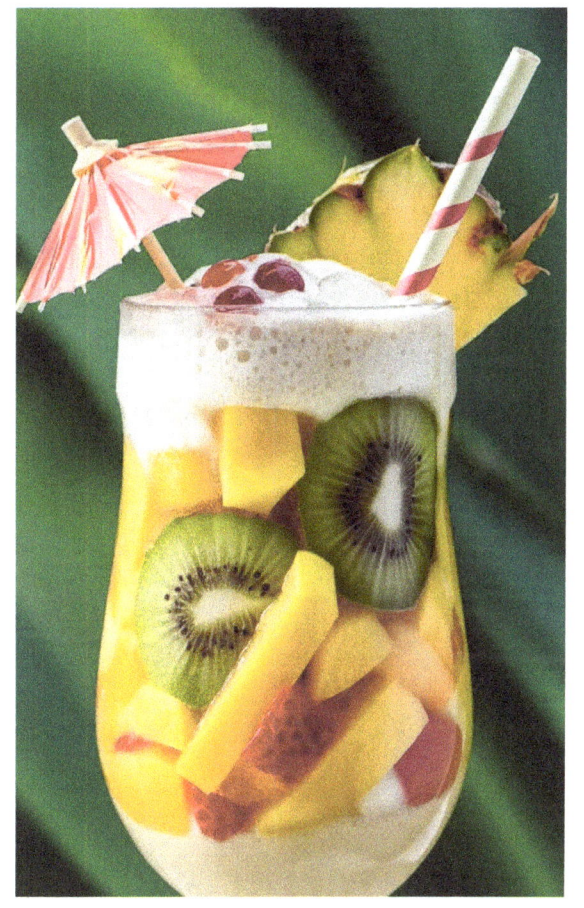

Instructions

- Place the frozen pineapple, mango, and banana chunks in a blender.
- Add the coconut water, Greek yogurt, honey (if using), and lime juice.
- Blend on high speed until smooth and creamy, adding more coconut water if necessary to reach your desired consistency.
- Pour into a glass and serve immediately.

Preparation Time : 5 min

Total Time : 5 min

Servings : 1

Nutritional Info

- Calories: 150
- Protein: 3g
- Carbohydrates: 35g
- Fat: 1g
- Fiber: 5g
- Sugar: 25g

BERRY PROTEIN SHAKE

Ingredients

- 1/2 cup mixed berries (strawberries, blueberries, raspberries)
- 1/2 cup unsweetened almond milk
- 1 scoop (about 30g) vanilla protein powder
- 1/4 cup plain Greek yogurt
- 1/2 banana, frozen
- 1/2 cup ice cubes

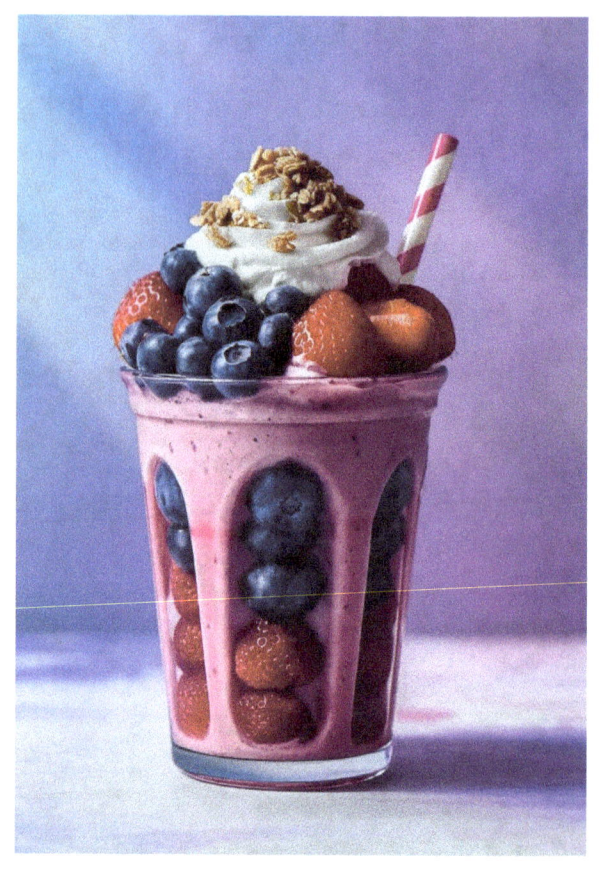

Instructions

- Add all ingredients to a blender.
- Blend on high speed until smooth and creamy, about 1-2 minutes.
- If the shake is too thick, add more almond milk, a little at a time, until desired consistency is reached.
- Pour into a glass and enjoy immediately!

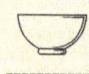 Preparation Time : 5 min

 Total Time : 5 min

 Servings : 1

Nutritional Info

- Calories: 200 kcal
- Protein: 20g
- Carbohydrates: 25g
- Fat: 2g
- Fiber: 5g

SPICED APPLE CIDER

Ingredients

- 6 medium apples, quartered (use a mix of sweet and tart varieties)
- 1 orange, sliced
- 3 cinnamon sticks
- 1 tablespoon whole cloves
- 1 tablespoon whole allspice berries
- 1 teaspoon ground nutmeg
- 8 cups water

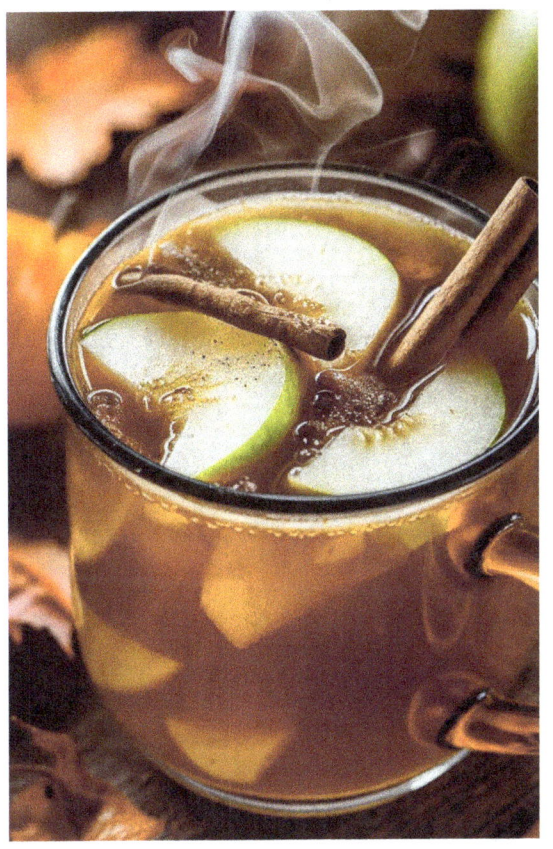

Instructions

- In a large pot, combine the quartered apples, orange slices, cinnamon sticks, whole cloves, whole allspice berries, ground nutmeg, and water.
- Bring the mixture to a boil over medium-high heat.
- Once boiling, reduce the heat to low and let the cider simmer for 30 minutes, uncovered, stirring occasionally.
- After 30 minutes, remove the pot from the heat and let it cool slightly.
- Using a fine mesh strainer or cheesecloth, strain the cider into a pitcher or another container to remove the solids.
- Serve the spiced apple cider warm, or refrigerate it for a few hours to serve chilled.
- Optionally, garnish each serving with a cinnamon stick or a slice of fresh apple.

 Preparation Time : 5 min

 Total Time : 35 min

 Servings : 4

Nutritional Info

- Calories: 60
- Total Fat: 0g
- Saturated Fat: 0g
- Cholesterol: 0mg
- Sodium: 5mg
- Total Carbohydrates: 16g

MATCHA GREEN TEA LATTE

Ingredients

- 1 teaspoon matcha green tea powder
- 1/4 cup hot water (not boiling)
- 3/4 cup unsweetened almond milk (or any milk of choice)
- 1-2 teaspoons honey or sweetener of choice (optional)

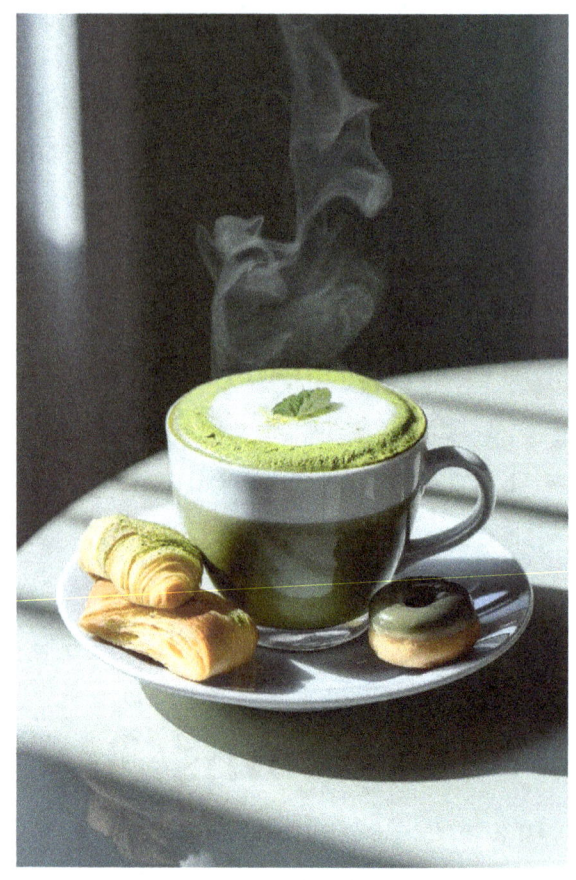

Instructions

- Prepare Matcha: Sift 1 teaspoon of matcha green tea powder into a mug to avoid clumps.
- Add Water: Pour 1/4 cup of hot water (not boiling) into the mug with the matcha powder. Whisk vigorously using a bamboo whisk or a small regular whisk until the matcha is fully dissolved and frothy.
- Heat Milk: In a small saucepan, heat 3/4 cup of unsweetened almond milk over medium heat until it is warm but not boiling. You can also heat the milk in the microwave for about 1-2 minutes.
- Combine: Pour the heated milk into the mug with the matcha mixture. Stir to combine.
- Sweeten (Optional): If desired, add 1-2 teaspoons of honey or your preferred sweetener and stir until dissolved.
- Serve: Enjoy your Matcha Green Tea Latte immediately while warm.

Preparation Time : 5 min

Total Time : 10 min

Servings : 1

Nutritional Info

- Calories: 40 (without sweetener)
- Protein: 1g
- Fat: 3g
- Carbohydrates: 2g
- Fiber: 1g
- Sugar: 0g (without sweetener)

GREEN DETOX SMOOTHIE

Ingredients

- 1 cup spinach, washed
- 1/2 cup kale, washed and stems removed
- 1/2 ripe avocado, peeled and pitted
- 1/2 banana, peeled
- 1/2 cup cucumber, peeled and chopped
- 1/2 cup unsweetened almond milk (or any milk of choice)
- Juice of 1/2 lemon
- 1 teaspoon grated ginger

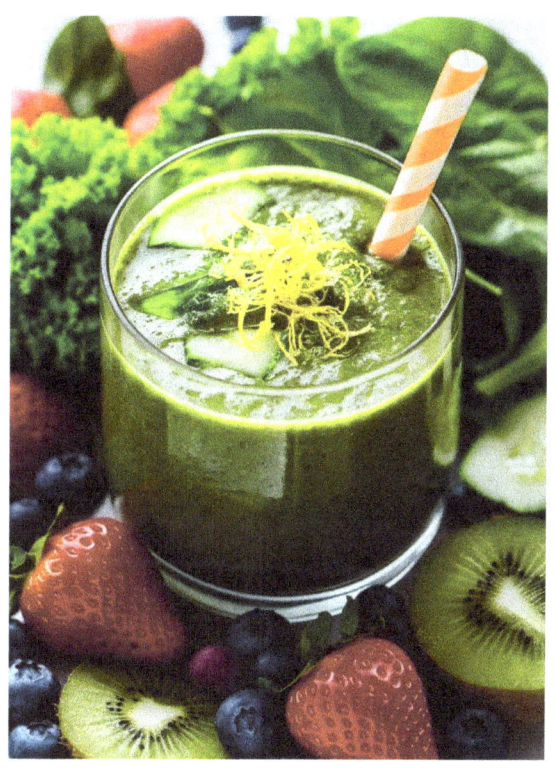

Instructions

- Place all the ingredients into a blender.
- Blend on high speed until smooth and creamy.
- If the smoothie is too thick, add more almond milk to reach your desired consistency.
- Taste and adjust sweetness by adding more banana if needed.
- Pour into a glass and enjoy immediately.

 Preparation Time : 5 min

 Total Time : 5 min

 Servings : 1

Nutritional Info

- Calories: 150 kcal
- Protein: 5g
- Carbohydrates: 25g
- Fat: 3g
- Fiber: 8g

HERBAL ICED TEA

Ingredients

- 1 herbal tea bag (such as chamomile, peppermint, or hibiscus)
- 1 cup water
- Ice cubes
- Optional: sweetener of your choice (honey, stevia, agave syrup)

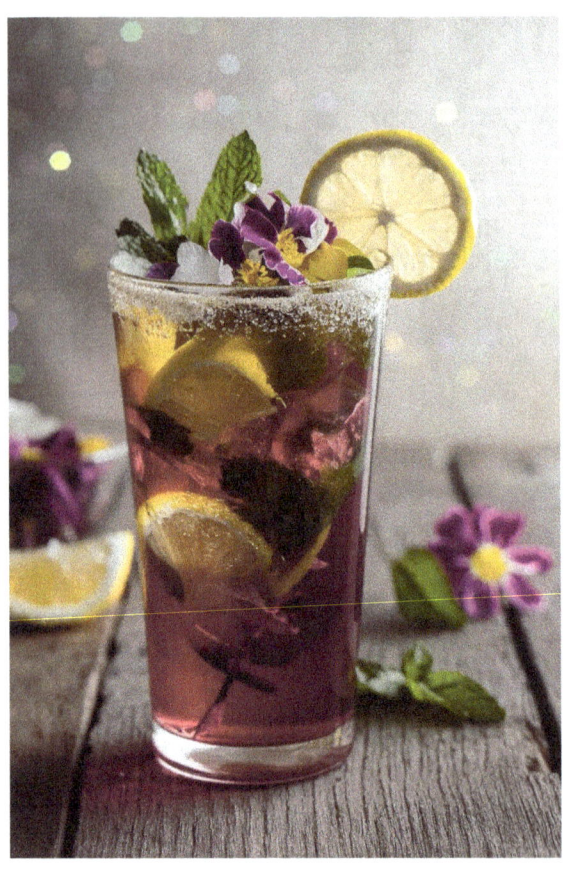

Instructions

- Boil 1 cup of water in a kettle or saucepan.
- Place the herbal tea bag in a heat-proof glass or mug.
- Pour the boiling water over the tea bag.
- Let the tea steep for 3-5 minutes, depending on your desired strength.
- Remove the tea bag and discard it.
- Allow the brewed tea to cool to room temperature.
- Once cooled, transfer the tea to a glass filled with ice cubes.
- Optionally, sweeten the tea with your preferred sweetener, stirring until dissolved.
- Garnish with a slice of lemon, a sprig of mint, or a slice of cucumber, if desired.
- Serve immediately and enjoy your refreshing Herbal Iced Tea!

Preparation Time : 5 min

Total Time : 5 min

Servings : 1

Nutritional Info

- Calories: 0 kcal
- Carbohydrates: 0 g
- Protein: 0 g
- Fat: 0 g
- Fiber: 0 g

BERRY LEMONADE

Ingredients

- 1 cup fresh strawberries, hulled and sliced
- 1 cup fresh blueberries
- 1 cup fresh raspberries
- 1 cup fresh blackberries
- 1 cup fresh lemon juice (about 4-6 lemons)
- 4 cups cold water
- 1-2 tablespoons honey or a natural sweetener (optional)
- Ice cubes
- Fresh mint leaves for garnish (optional)

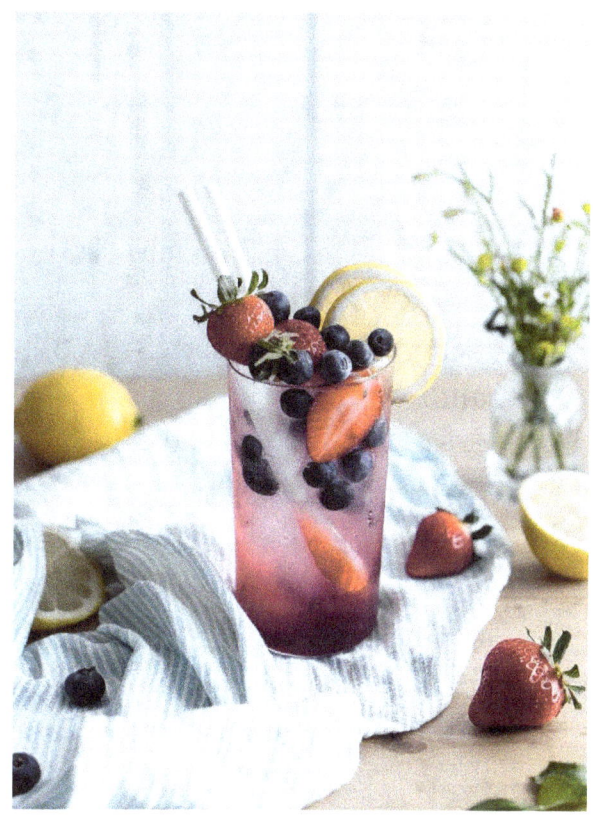

Instructions

- Wash the strawberries, blueberries, raspberries, and blackberries thoroughly.
- Hull and slice the strawberries.
- Place the strawberries, blueberries, raspberries, and blackberries in a blender.
- Blend until smooth.
- Pour the blended berry mixture through a fine mesh sieve or cheesecloth into a large pitcher to remove seeds and pulp. Use a spoon to press the mixture through the sieve if needed.
- Add the freshly squeezed lemon juice to the pitcher.
- Pour in the cold water and stir well.
- If desired, add honey or your preferred natural sweetener to the pitcher and stir until dissolved.
- Fill glasses with ice cubes.
- Pour the berry lemonade over the ice.
- Garnish with fresh mint leaves if desired.
- Serve immediately and enjoy your refreshing berry lemonade!

 Preparation Time : 15 min

 Total Time : 15 min

 Servings : 4

Nutritional Info

- Calories: 50
- Protein: 1g
- Carbohydrates: 13g
- Dietary Fiber: 4g
- Sugars: 9g
- Fat: 0g

Shopping List for Psoriasis-Friendly Foods

Fresh Produce
- **Leafy Greens:** Spinach, kale, Swiss chard, arugula
- **Cruciferous Vegetables:** Broccoli, cauliflower, Brussels sprouts
- **Berries:** Blueberries, strawberries, raspberries, blackberries
- **Other Vegetables:** Carrots, sweet potatoes, bell peppers, cucumbers
- **Fruits:** Apples, oranges, avocados, bananas

Proteins
- **Lean Meats:** Chicken breast, turkey breast
- **Fatty Fish:** Salmon, mackerel, sardines, trout
- **Plant-Based Proteins:** Tofu, legumes (black beans, chickpeas, lentils)

Whole Grains
- **Grains:** Brown rice, quinoa, barley, oats
- **Whole Wheat:** Whole wheat bread, whole wheat pasta

Healthy Fats
- **Oils:** Extra virgin olive oil, avocado oil, coconut oil
- **Nuts and Seeds:** Almonds, walnuts, flaxseeds, chia seeds, sunflower seeds

Dairy and Alternatives
- **Dairy Alternatives:** Almond milk, coconut milk, soy milk
- **Yoghurt:** Greek yoghurt (preferably unsweetened, for those who can tolerate dairy)

Fermented Foods
- **Fermented Vegetables:** Sauerkraut, kimchi
- **Fermented Dairy:** Kefir (non-dairy options available)

Snacks
- **Healthy Snacks:** Dried fruit (unsweetened), seaweed snacks, rice cakes

Herbs and Spices
- **Anti-inflammatory Spices:** Turmeric, ginger, garlic powder, cinnamon
- **Fresh Herbs:** Basil, oregano, parsley, cilantro

Beverages
- **Teas:** Green tea, herbal teas
- **Hydration:** Coconut water

Condiments
- **Healthy Condiments:** Apple cider vinegar, tahini, low sodium soy sauce or tamari, mustard

Miscellaneous
- **Canned Goods:** Tuna, salmon (in water), diced tomatoes, artichoke hearts
- **Other:** Olives, capers

Sleep Hygiene and Skin Health

Importance

1. **Cell Regeneration:** During sleep, the body repairs and regenerates skin cells. Adequate sleep allows for proper healing and rejuvenation, which is essential for managing skin conditions like psoriasis.
2. **Inflammation Reduction**: Poor sleep can lead to increased inflammation in the body. Since psoriasis is an inflammatory condition, getting enough rest can help reduce flare-ups and manage symptoms.
3. **Hormonal Balance:** Sleep affects the balance of various hormones in the body, including those that regulate stress. Stress can exacerbate psoriasis, so good sleep hygiene can help maintain hormonal balance and reduce stress levels.
4. **Immune Function:** Adequate sleep supports a healthy immune system. Since psoriasis is an autoimmune condition, a well-functioning immune system can help keep symptoms under control.

Tips for Better Sleep Hygiene

1. **Consistent Sleep Schedule:** Go to bed and wake up at the same time every day, even on weekends. This helps regulate your body's internal clock.
2. **Create a Relaxing Bedtime Routine**: Establish a calming pre-sleep routine. Activities like reading, taking a warm bath, or practising meditation can signal to your body that it's time to wind down.
3. **Comfortable Sleep Environment:** Ensure your bedroom is conducive to sleep. This includes a comfortable mattress and pillows, a cool temperature, and minimal noise and light.
4. **Limit Screen Time**: Reduce exposure to screens (phones, tablets, TVs) at least an hour before bed. The blue light emitted by screens can interfere with your body's production of _melatonin_, a hormone that regulates sleep.
5. **Avoid Stimulants:** Limit consumption of caffeine and nicotine, especially in the hours leading up to bedtime. These stimulants can disrupt sleep patterns.

Natural Remedies and Supplements

1. **Aloe Vera**
- **Use**: Apply aloe vera gel directly to the skin.
- **Benefits**: Helps soothe and moisturize the skin, reducing redness and scaling.

2. **Apple Cider Vinegar**
- **Use**: Dilute with water and apply to the scalp or skin.
- **Benefits**: Can help relieve itching and scaling, especially on the scalp.

3. **Oatmeal Baths**
- **Use**: Add colloidal oatmeal to a warm bath and soak for 15-20 minutes.
- **Benefits**: Soothes itching and softens the skin.

4. **Dead Sea Salt Baths**
- **Use**: Dissolve Dead Sea salts in a warm bath and soak for 15-20 minutes.
- **Benefits**: Helps to improve skin hydration and reduce inflammation.

5. **Tea Tree Oil**
- **Use**: Dilute with a carrier oil (like coconut or olive oil) and apply to the affected areas.
- **Benefits**: Has anti-inflammatory and antimicrobial properties that can help reduce flare-ups.

Supplements

1. **Fish Oil (Omega-3 Fatty Acids)**
- **Use**: Take fish oil supplements as directed.
- **Benefits**: Reduces inflammation and improves skin health. Found in fatty fish like salmon, mackerel, and sardines.

2. **Vitamin D**
- **Use**: Take vitamin D supplements or increase exposure to sunlight.
- **Benefits**: Helps modulate the immune system and reduce psoriasis symptoms.

3. **Probiotics**
- **Use**: Take probiotic supplements or eat fermented foods like yoghurt, kefir, sauerkraut, and kimchi.
- **Benefits**: Supports gut health, which can influence immune response and inflammation.

4. **Aloe Vera Capsules**
- **Use**: Take aloe vera supplements as directed.
- **Benefits**: Supports skin healing and reduces inflammation.

5. **Milk Thistle**
- **Use**: Take milk thistle supplements as directed.
- **Benefits**: Detoxifies the liver, which can help manage psoriasis symptoms.

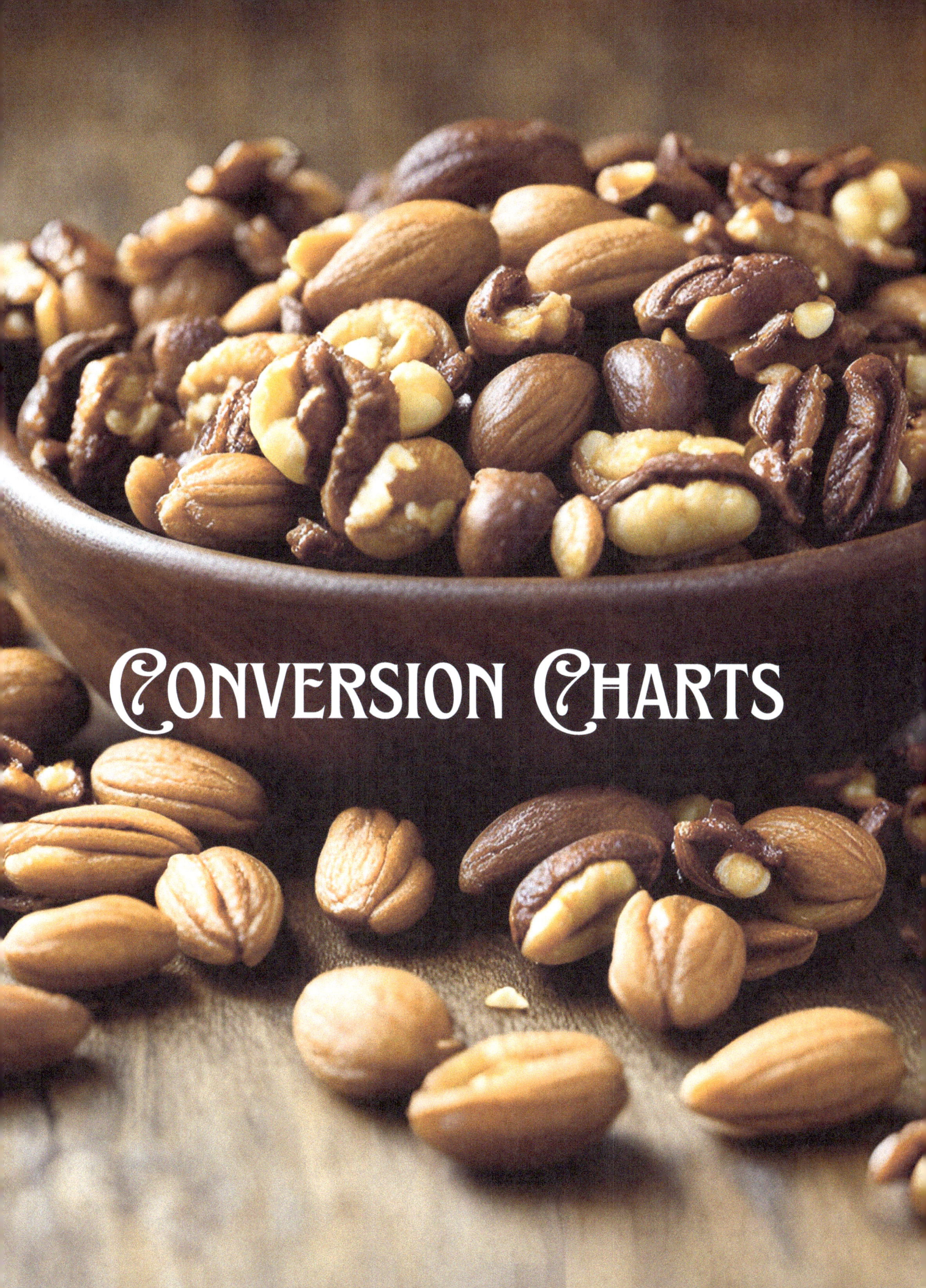

Conversion Charts

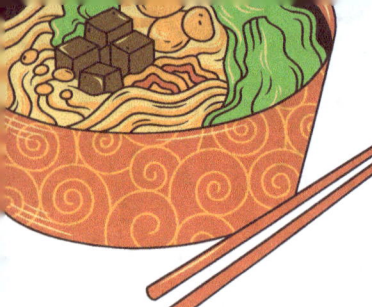
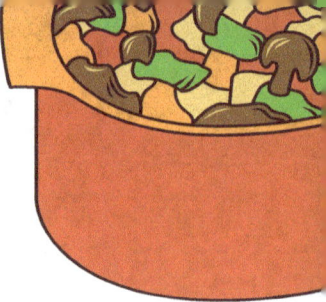

COMMON COOKING MEASUREMENTS

Volume Measurements

MEASUREMENT	EQUIVALENT
1 teaspoon (tsp)	1/3 tablespoon (tbsp)
1 teaspoon (tsp)	3 teaspoons (tsp)
1/8 cup	2 tablespoons (tbsp)
1/4 cup	4 tablespoons (tbsp)
1/3 cup	5 tablespoons + 1 teaspoon
1/2 cup	8 tablespoons (tbsp)
3/4 cup	12 tablespoons (tbsp)
1 cup	16 tablespoons (tbsp)
1 pint (pt)	2 cups
1 quart (qt)	4 cups
1 gallon (gal)	16 cups

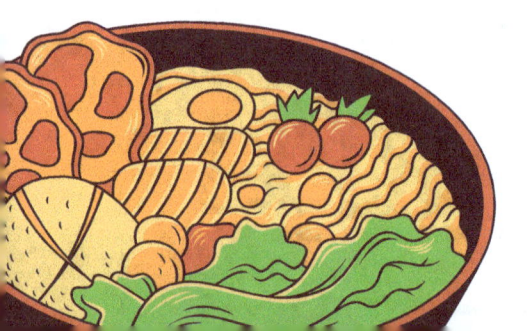
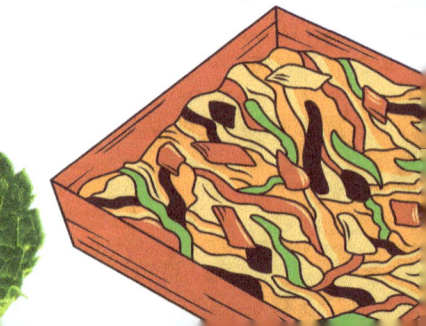

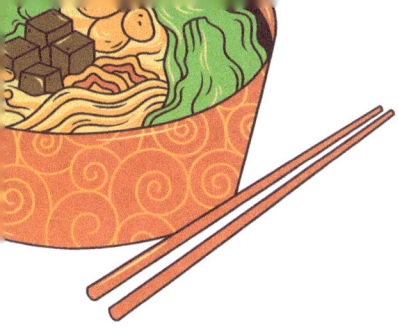
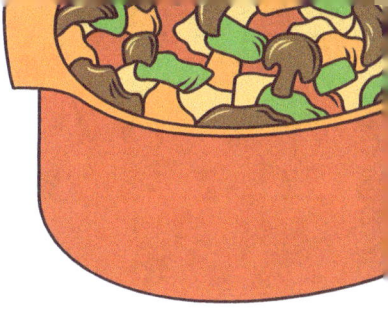

Weight Measurements

MEASUREMENT	EQUIVALENT
1 ounce (oz)	28.35 grams (g)
1 pound (lb)	16 ounces (oz)
1 kilogram (kg)	2.2 pounds (lbs)

Liquid Measurements

MEASUREMENT	EQUIVALENT
1 fluid ounce (fl oz)	2 tablespoons (tbsp)
1 cup	8 fluid ounces (fl oz)
1 pint (pt)	16 fluid ounces (fl oz)
1 quart (qt)	32 fluid ounces (fl oz)
1 gallon (gal)	128 fluid ounces (fl oz)

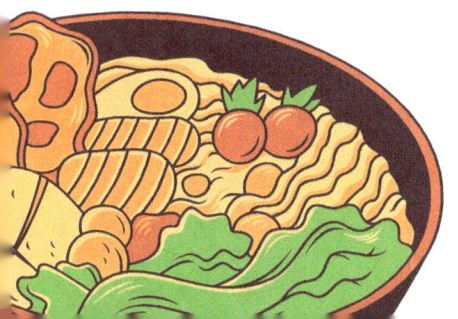
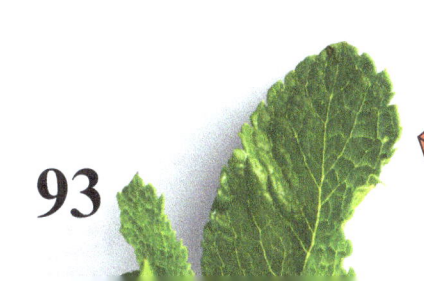
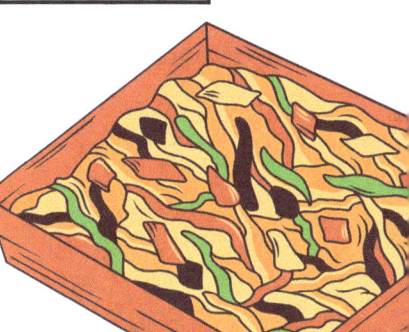

OVEN TEMPERATURES
Temperature Conversions

FAHRENHEIT (°F)	CELSIUS (°C)	GAS MARK
250°F	120°C	1/2
275°F	135°C	1
300°F	150°C	2
325°F	165°C	3
350°F	175°C	4
375°F	190°C	5
400°F	200°C	6
425°F	220°C	7
450°F	230°C	8
475°F	245°C	9
500°F	260°C	10

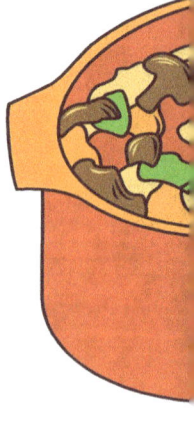
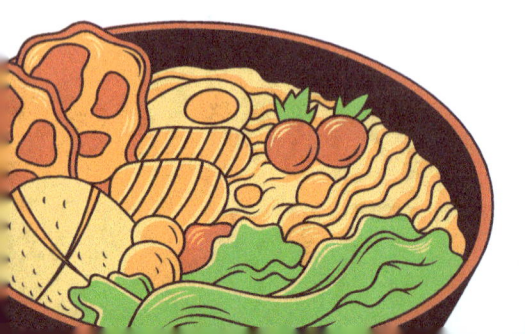

METRIC CONVERSIONS

Volume

METRIC	U.S. EQUIVALENT
1 milliliter (ml)	0.034 fluid ounces (fl oz)
100 milliliters	3.4 fluid ounces (fl oz)
1 liter (l)	34 fluid ounces (fl oz)
1 liter (l)	4.2 cups
1 liter (l)	2.1 pints

Weight

METRIC	U.S. EQUIVALENT
1 gram (g)	0.035 ounces (oz)
100 grams (g)	3.5 ounces (oz)
500 grams (g)	17.6 ounces (oz)
1 kilogram (kg)	2.2 pounds (lbs)

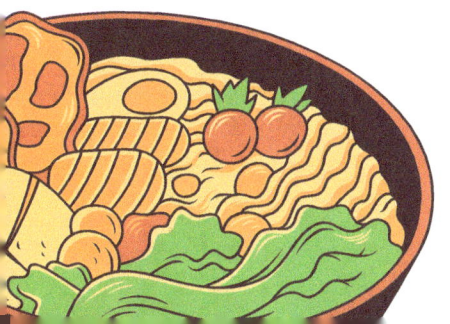
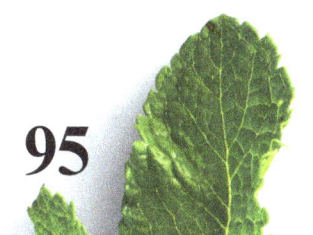
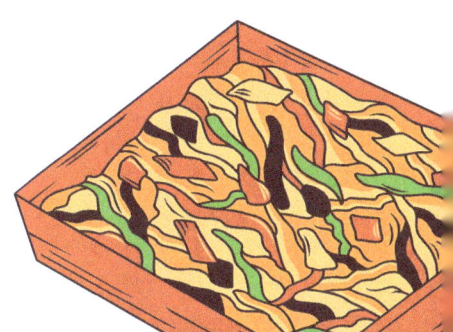

Conclusion

As we come to the end of this journey through the "Psoriasis Diet for Beginners," I hope that you feel empowered and inspired to take control of your health through the choices you make every day. This cookbook has been more than just a collection of recipes; it's a guide to embracing a lifestyle that nourishes your body, soothes your skin, and uplifts your spirit.

Psoriasis is a challenging condition, but it doesn't define you. By incorporating the dietary strategies and lifestyle tips shared in this book, you are taking proactive steps towards managing your symptoms and improving your quality of life. The foods you eat can have a profound impact on your skin health, and with the right ingredients and recipes, you can enjoy delicious meals while supporting your body's healing processes.

Remember, every person's journey with psoriasis is unique. What works for one might not work for another, and it's okay to experiment and find what suits you best. Keep a positive mindset, stay patient, and celebrate every small victory along the way.

The recipes and tips in this book are just the beginning. They are a foundation upon which you can build a healthier, more vibrant life. Continue to explore, learn, and adapt. Listen to your body, honor its needs, and never underestimate the power of good nutrition and self-care.

As you move forward, I encourage you to stay connected with a supportive community, seek advice from healthcare professionals, and remain informed about new advancements in psoriasis management. The path to wellness is ongoing, but with each step you take, you are closer to achieving balance and harmony within your body.

Thank you for allowing me to be a part of your journey. May your kitchen be filled with the aromas of healing foods, your table be a place of joy and togetherness, and your heart be full of hope and determination. Here's to a healthier, happier you, one delicious meal at a time.

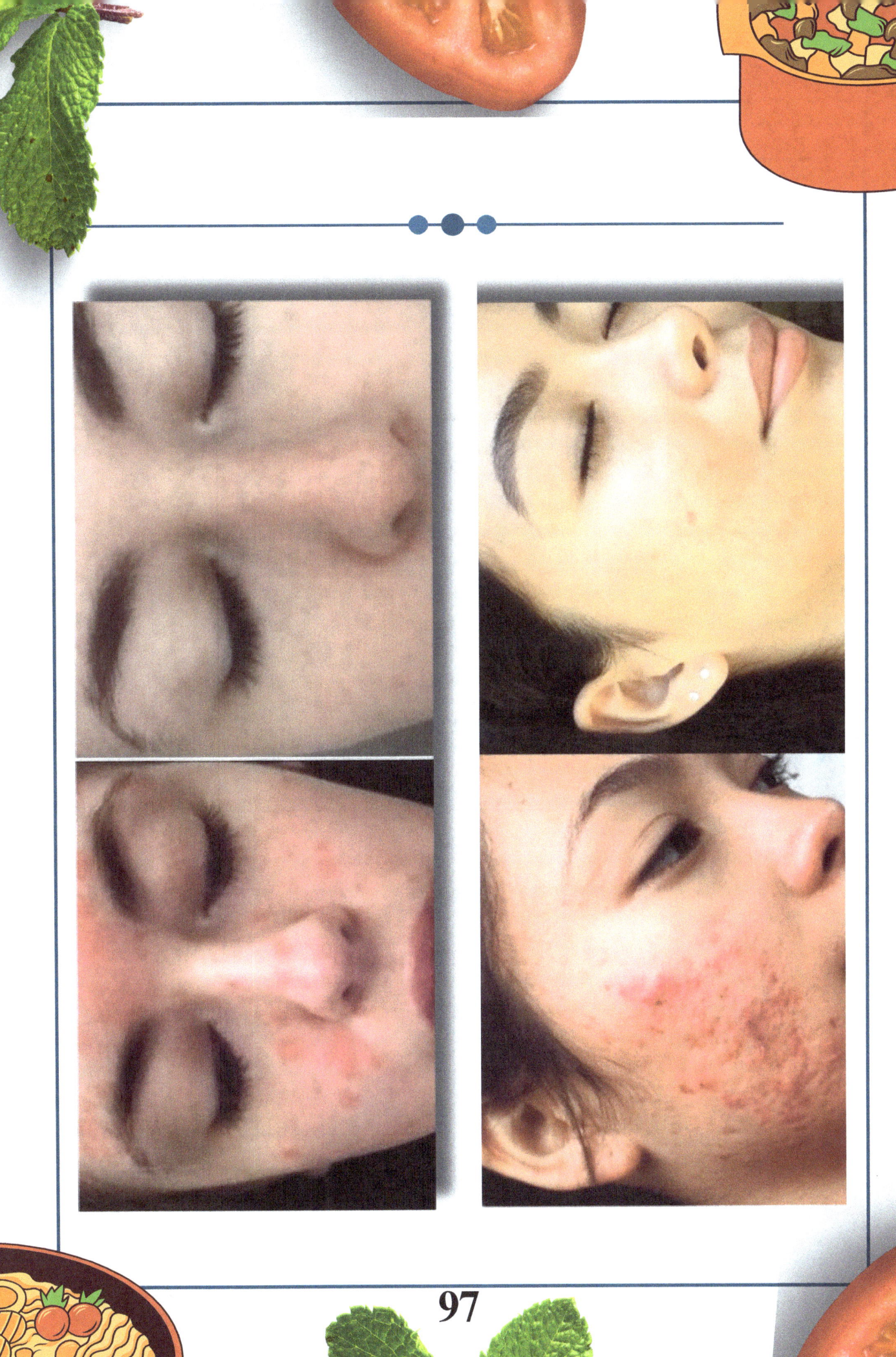

DISCOVER MORE ABOUT MY CULINARY ADVENTURES AND UPCOMING PROJECTS.

About
THE AUTHOR

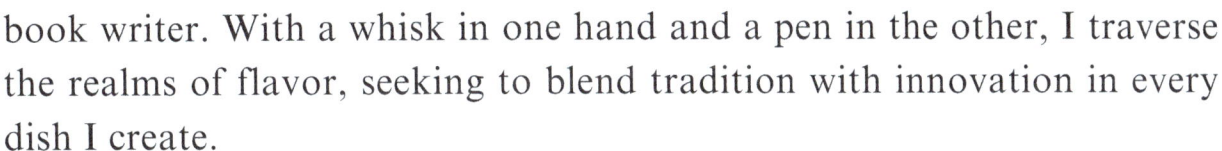

Hello, culinary adventurers! I'm Vakare Rimkute, a passionate explorer of the culinary world and a devoted recipe book writer. With a whisk in one hand and a pen in the other, I traverse the realms of flavor, seeking to blend tradition with innovation in every dish I create.

Growing up in the bustling kitchens of my Lithuanian grandmother, I developed an insatiable curiosity for the alchemy of ingredients and the magic they could weave on the palate. From the rustic charm of hearty stews to the delicate intricacies of pastries, my journey through food has been nothing short of a delightful adventure.

After years of experimenting and honing my craft, I found my true calling as a recipe book writer. With each recipe I pen, I aim to capture the essence of culinary culture while infusing it with a touch of modern flair. From comforting classics to bold culinary experiments, my recipes are a reflection of my belief that food should not only nourish the body but also nourish the soul.

So join me on this gastronomic journey, where every page is filled with tantalizing flavors, heartwarming stories, and a dash of humor. Together, let's embark on a culinary adventure that will tickle your taste buds and leave you craving for more. Happy cooking!

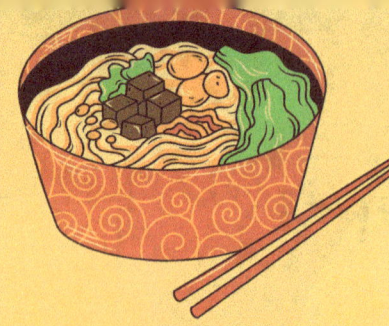
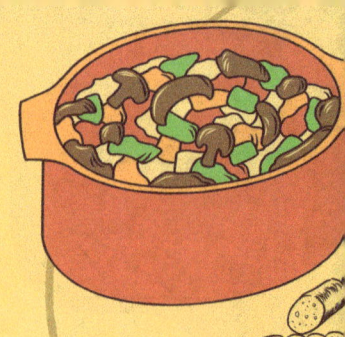

My Weekly Meal Planner

DAY	BREAKFAST	LUNCH	DINNER
MONDAY			
TUESDAY			
WEDNESDAY			
THURSDAY			
FRIDAY			
SATURDAY			
SUNDAY			

@REALLYGREATSITE

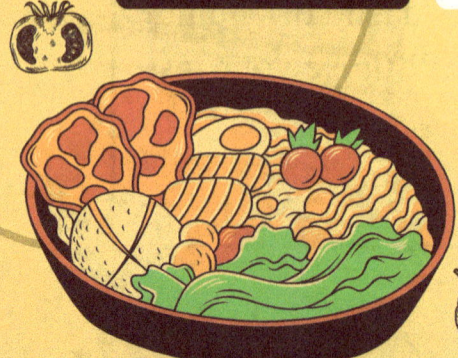
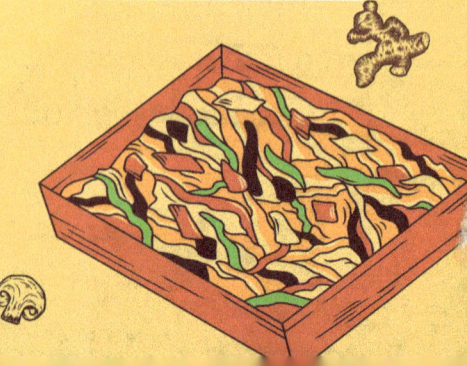

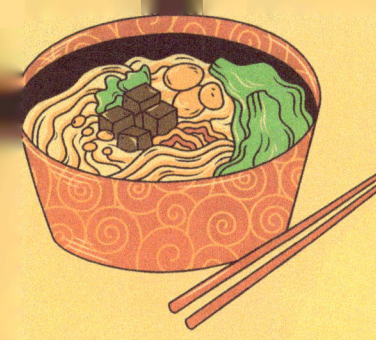
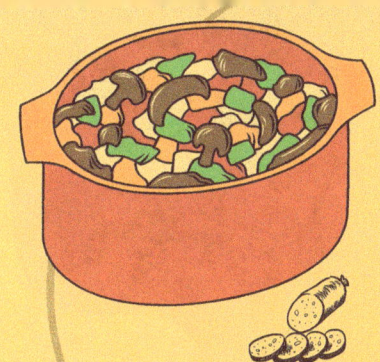

My Weekly Meal Planner

DAY	BREAKFAST	LUNCH	DINNER
MONDAY			
TUESDAY			
WEDNESDAY			
THURSDAY			
FRIDAY			
SATURDAY			
SUNDAY			

@REALLYGREATSITE

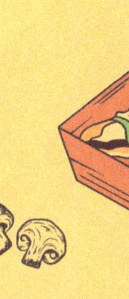
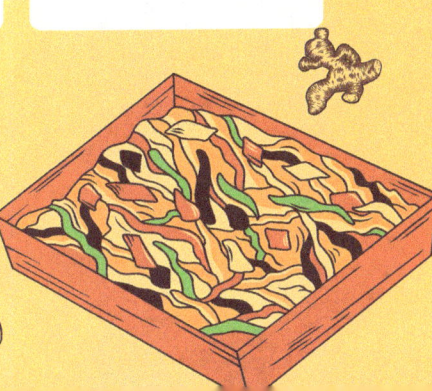

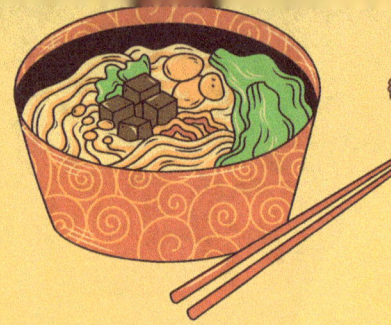
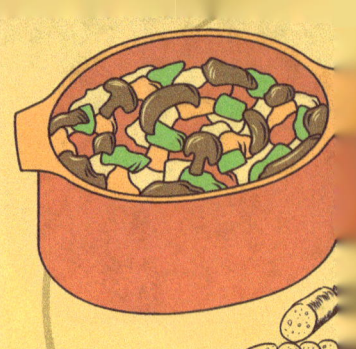

My Weekly Meal Planner

DAY	BREAKFAST	LUNCH	DINNER
MONDAY			
TUESDAY			
WEDNESDAY			
THURSDAY			
FRIDAY			
SATURDAY			
SUNDAY			

@REALLYGREATSITE

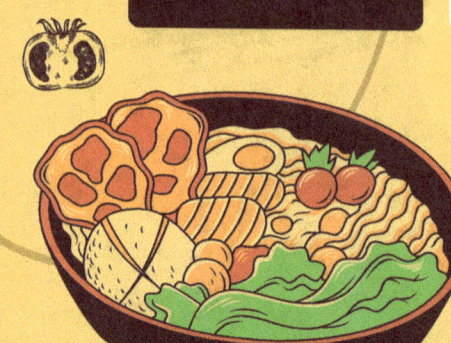
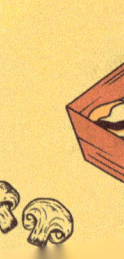
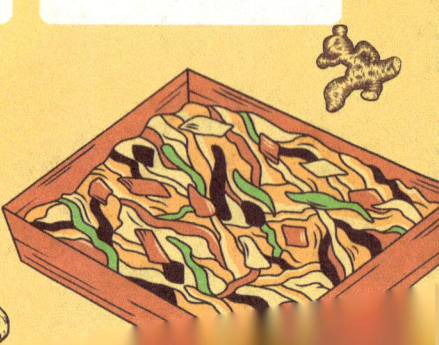

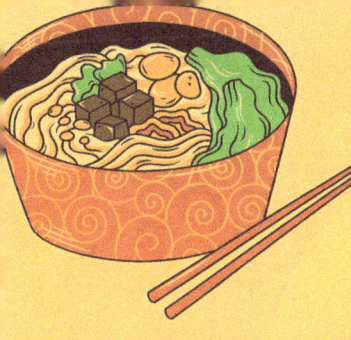
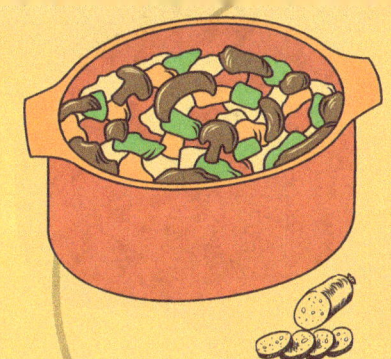

My Weekly Meal Planner

DAY	BREAKFAST	LUNCH	DINNER
MONDAY			
TUESDAY			
WEDNESDAY			
THURSDAY			
FRIDAY			
SATURDAY			
SUNDAY			

@REALLYGREATSITE

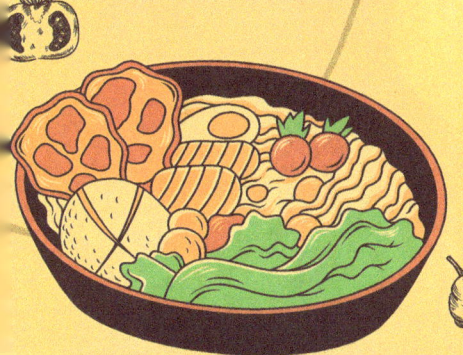
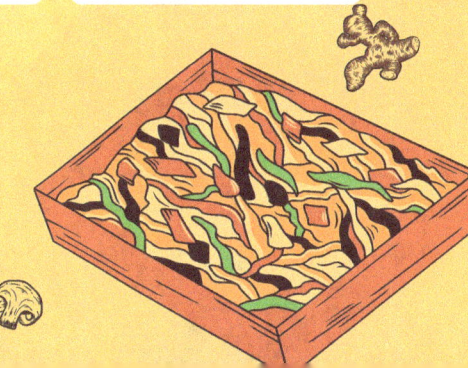

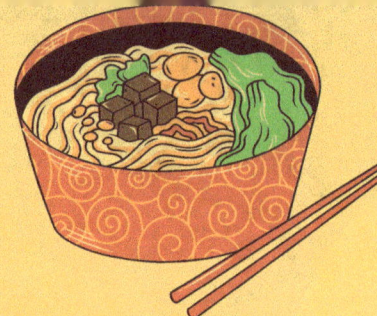
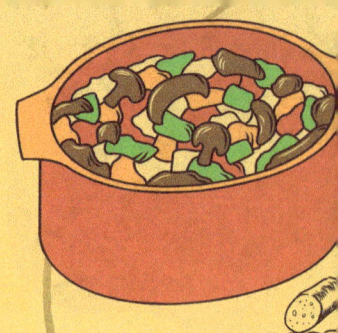

My Weekly Meal Planner

DAY	BREAKFAST	LUNCH	DINNER
MONDAY			
TUESDAY			
WEDNESDAY			
THURSDAY			
FRIDAY			
SATURDAY			
SUNDAY			

@REALLYGREATSITE

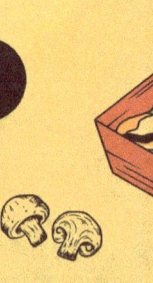
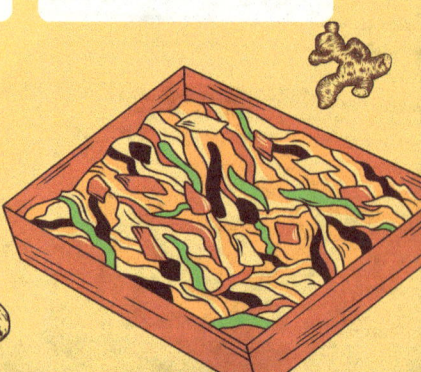

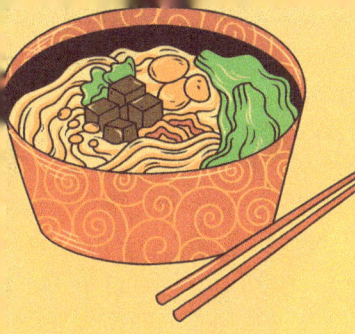
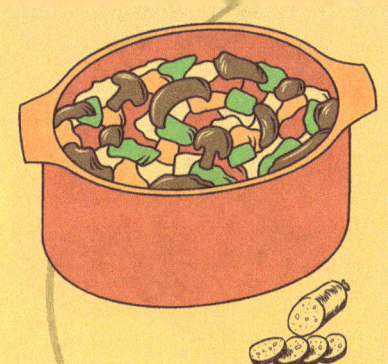

My Weekly Meal Planner

DAY	BREAKFAST	LUNCH	DINNER
MONDAY			
TUESDAY			
WEDNESDAY			
THURSDAY			
FRIDAY			
SATURDAY			
SUNDAY			

@REALLYGREATSITE

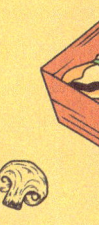
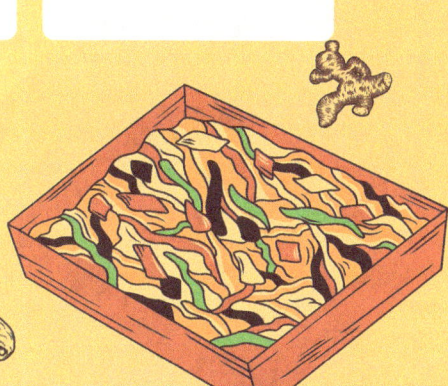

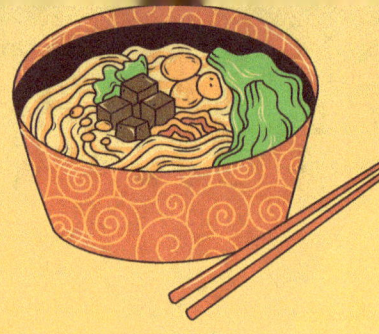
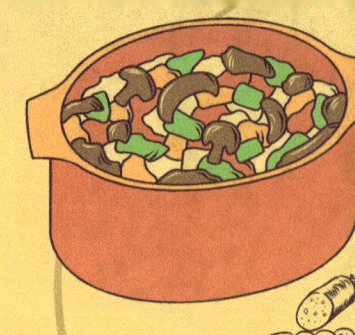

My Weekly Meal Planner

DAY	BREAKFAST	LUNCH	DINNER
MONDAY			
TUESDAY			
WEDNESDAY			
THURSDAY			
FRIDAY			
SATURDAY			
SUNDAY			

@REALLYGREATSITE

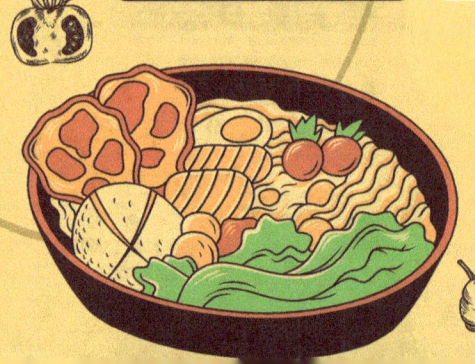
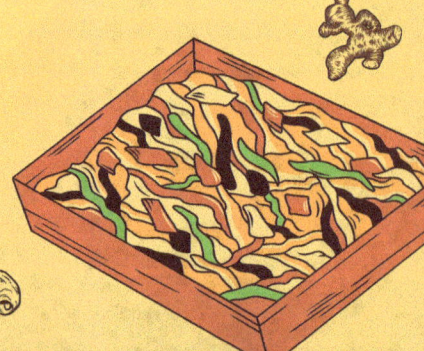

www.ingramcontent.com/pod-product-compliance
Lightning Source LLC
Chambersburg PA
CBHW062314220526
45479CB00004B/1160